T0320558

MONOCLONAL ANTIBODY THERAPY
OF HUMAN CANCER

DEVELOPMENTS IN ONCOLOGY

F.J. Cleton and J.W.I.M. Simons, eds.: Genetic Origins of Tumour Cells. 90-247-2272-1.
J. Aisner and P. Chang, eds.: Cancer Treatment and Research. 90-247-2358-2.
B.W. Ongerboer de Visser, D.A. Bosch and W.M.H. van Woerkom-Eykenboom, eds.: Neuro-oncology: Clinical and Experimental Aspects. 90-247-2421-X.
K. Hellmann, P. Hilgard and S. Eccles, eds.: Metastasis: Clinical and Experimental Aspects. 90-247-2424-4.
H.F. Seigler, ed.: Clinical Management of Melanoma. 90-247-2584-4.
P. Correa and W. Haenszel, eds.: Epidemiology of Cancer of the Digestive Tract. 90-247-2601-8.
L.A. Liotta and I.R. Hart, eds.: Tumour Invasion and Metastasis. 90-247-2611-5.
J. Banoczy, ed.: Oral Leukoplakia. 90-247-2655-7.
C. Tijssen, M. Halprin and L. Endtz, eds.: Familial Brain Tumours. 90-247-2691-3.
F.M. Muggia, C.W. Young and S.K. Carter, eds.: Anthracycline Antibiotics in Cancer. 90-247-2711-1
B.W. Hancock, ed.: Assessment of Tumour Response. 90-247-2712-X.
D.E. Peterson, ed.: Oral Complications of Cancer Chemotherapy. 0-89838-563-6.
R. Mastrangelo, D.G. Poplack and R. Riccardi, eds.: Central Nervous System Leukemia. Prevention and Treatment. 0-89838-570-9.
A. Polliack, ed.: Human Leukemias. Cytochemical and Ultrastructural Techniques in Diagnosis and Research. 0-89838-585-7.
W. Davis, C. Maltoni and S. Tanneberger, eds.: The Control of Tumor Growth and its Biological Bases 0-89838-603-9.
A.P.M. Heintz, C. Th. Griffiths and J.B. Trimbos, eds.: Surgery in Gynecological Oncology. 0-89838-604-7.
M.P. Hacker, E.B. Douple and I. Krakoff, eds.: Platinum Coordination Complexes in Cancer Chemotherapy. 0-89838-619-5.
M.J. van Zwieten. The Rat as Animal Model in Breast Cancer Research: A Histopathological Study c Radiation- and Hormone-Induced Rat Mammary Tumors. 0-89838-624-1.
B. Lowenberg and A. Hogenbeck, eds.: Minimal Residual Disease in Acute Leukemia. 0-89838-630-6
I. van der Waal and G.B. Snow, eds.: Oral Oncology. 0-89838-631-4.
B.W. Hancock and A.M. Ward, eds.: Immunological Aspects of Cancer. 0-89838-664-0.
K.V. Honn and B.F. Sloane, eds.: Hemostatic Mechanisms and Metastasis. 0-89838-667-5.
K.R. Harrap, W. Davis and A.N. Calvert, eds.: Cancer Chemotherapy and Selective Drug Development. 0-89838-673-X.
V.D. Velde, J.H. Cornelis and P.H. Sugarbaker, eds.: Liver Metastasis. 0-89838-648-5.
D.J. Ruiter, K. Welvaart and S. Ferrone, eds.: Cutaneous Melanoma and Precursor Lesions. 0-89838-689-6.
S.B. Howell, ed.: Intra-Arterial and Intracavitary Cancer Chemotherapy. 0-89838-691-8.
D.L. Kisner and J.F. Smyth, eds.: Interferon Alpha-2: Pre-Clinical and Clinical Evaluation. 0-89838-701-9.
P. Furmanski, J.C. Hager and M.A. Rich, eds.: RNA Tumor Viruses, Oncogenes, Human Cancer ar Aids: On the Frontiers of Understanding. 0-89838-703-5.
J.E. Talmadge, I.J. Fidler and R.K. Oldham: Screening for Biological Response Modifiers: Methods and Rationale. 0-89838-712-4.
J.C. Bottino, R.W. Opfell and F.M. Muggia, eds.: Liver Cancer. 0-89838-713-2.
P.K. Pattengale, R.J. Lukes and C.R. Taylor, eds.: Lymphoproliferative Diseases: Pathogenesis, Diagnosis, Therapy. 0-89838-725-6.
F. Cavalli, G. Bonadonna and M. Rozencweig, eds.: Malignant Lymphomas and Hodgkin's Disease. 0-89838-727-2.
L. Baker, F. Valeriote and V. Ratanatharathorn, eds.: Biology and Therapy of Acute Leukemi' 0-89838-728-0.
J. Russo, ed.: Immunocytochemistry in Tumor Diagnosis. 0-89838-737-X.
R.L. Ceriani, ed.: Monoclonal Antibodies and Breast Cancer. 0-89838-739-6.
D.E. Peterson, G.E. Elias and S.T. Sonis, eds.: Head and Neck Management of the Cancer Patier 0-89838-747-7.
D.M. Green: Diagnosis and Management of Malignant Solid Tumors in Infants and Children. 0-89838-750-7.

MONOCLONAL ANTIBODY THERAPY OF HUMAN CANCER

edited by

Kenneth A. Foon
Simpson Memorial Research Institute
University of Michigan, Ann Arbor

and

Alton C. Morgan, Jr.
NeoRx, Inc.
Seattle, Washington

Martinus Nijhoff Publishing
a member of the Kluwer Academic Publishers Group
Boston/Dordrecht/Lancaster

Distributors for North America:
Kluwer Academic Publishers
190 Old Derby Street
Hingham, MA 02043, USA

Distributors for the UK and Ireland:
Kluwer Academic Publishers
MTP Press Limited
Falcon House, Queen Square
Lancaster LA1 1RN, UNITED KINGDOM

Distributors for all other countries:
Kluwer Academic Publishers Group
Distribution Centre
P.O. Box 322
3300 AH Dordrecht, THE NETHERLANDS

Library of Congress Cataloging in Publication Data
Main entry under title:

Monoclonal antibody therapy of human cancer.

(Developments in oncology)
Includes bibliographies and index.
1. Antibodies, Monoclonal—Therapeutic use.
2. Cancer—Treatment. 3. Immunotherapy. I. Foon,
Kenneth A. II. Morgan, Alton C. III. Series.
[DNLM: 1. Antibodies, Monoclonal—therapeutic use.
2. Neoplasms—therapy. W1 DE998N / QZ 266 M7513]
RC271.M65M66 1985   616.99′406   85–15406
ISBN 0–89838–754–X

Printed in the United States of America

CONTENTS

CONTRIBUTORS

PAUL G. ABRAMS, M.D.
Vice President & Medical Director
NeoRx, Inc.
410 West Harrison Street
Seattle, Washington 98119

R. W. BALDWIN, PH.D., F.R.C. PATH.
Director, Cancer Research Campaign Laboratories
The University
Nottingham
NG7 2RD
United Kingdom

PAUL A. BUNN, M.D.
Chief, Division of Medical Oncology
University of Colorado
Health Sciences Center
Box B171
4200 East 9th Avenue
Denver, Colorado 80262

KENNETH A. FOON, M.D.
Assoc. Dir., Div. of Hematology/Oncology
University of Michigan
Simpson Memorial Research Institute
102 Observatory
Ann Arbor, Michigan 48109

KOU M. HWANG, PH.D.
Professor, Department of Pharmacology
Rutgers University
New Brunswick, New Jersey 08903

STEVEN M. LARSON, M.D.
Chief, Nuclear Medicine Department
National Institutes of Health
9000 Rockville Pike
Building 10, Room 1C401
Bethesda, Maryland 20205

CAROL L. MACLEOD, PH.D.
Assistant Professor
Department of Medicine
Cancer Center, T-011
University of California
   at San Diego
La Jolla, California 92093

HIDEO MASUI, PH.D.
Associate Research Biologist
Cancer Center, T-011
University of California
  at San Diego
La Jolla, California 92093

JOHN MENDELSOHN, M.D.
Chief of Medicine
Memorial Sloan-Kettering Cancer Center
1275 York Avenue
New York, New York 10021

ALTON C. MORGAN, JR., PH.D.
Scientific Director of Tumor Immunology
NeoRx, Inc.
410 West Harrison Street
Seattle, Washington 98119

ROBERT K. OLDHAM, M.D.
Director, Biological Therapy Institute
Riverside Drive
Franklin, Tennessee 37064

GOWSALA PAVANASASIVAM, PH.D.
Head, Immunoconjugate Section
NeoRx, Inc.
410 West Harrison Street
Seattle, Washington 98119

ROBERT W. SCHROFF, PH.D.
Head, Immunologic Assessment Section
NeoRx, Inc.
410 West Harrison Street
Seattle, Washington 98119

HENRY C. STEVENSON, M.D.
Senior Investigator
Clinical Investigations Section
Biological Response Modifiers Program
National Cancer Institute
Frederick, Maryland 21701

IAN S. TROWBRIDGE, PH.D.
Senior Member
Department of Cancer Biology
The Salk Institute
San Diego, California 92138

JAMES M. WOOLFENDEN, M.D.
Department of Radiology
Division of Nuclear Medicine
College of Medicine
University of Arizona
Tucson, Arizona 85724

PREFACE

KENNETH A. FOON and ALTON C. MORGAN, JR.

Passive immunotherapy using heteroantisera for the treatment of cancer in animals and humans has been studied for over 50 years. Attempts have been made to treat animal tumors with sera from immunized syngeneic, allogeneic, or xenogeneic animals. A number of studies of passive immunotherapy using heterologous antisera in humans have also been performed. These studies have generally been attempted in patients with large tumor burdens, and as would be expected, results have been transient at best. A wide variety of solid tumors as well as leukemias and lymphomas have been treated with antisera raised in sheep, horses, rabbits, and goats. Problems such as anaphylaxis, serum sickness, and severe cytopenias have been encountered with these antisera.

There are a number of potential mechanisms by which unconjugated antibodies might be cytotoxic to tumor cells. Antibodies bound to the cell surface membrane of tumor cells may lead to cell lysis by complement-dependent or antibody-dependent cellular cytotoxicity. Circulating tumor cells bound by antibody may be more susceptible to phagocytosis by the reticuloendothelial system. Antibody bound to the cell surface membrane of tumor cells may enhance immunogenicity of the tumor cell leading to activation of the host's immune system. In any of these cases, successful therapy with antibodies is dependent on the accessibility of the antibody to the tumor, the density and heterogeneity of antigen expression by the tumor, the natural immunity of the host, the degree of specificity of the antibodies used for targeting, and the class of antibody injected.

Due to the potential for targeting of cytotoxic agents, attempts have been made to link tumor-specific heteroantisera to drugs such as methotrexate, chlorambucil, and daunorubicin. Other agents such as radioisotopes, toxins, and enzymes have also been conjugated to antibody. One of the major problems encountered in these initial attempts at immunoconjugate preparation has been the inability to develop tumor-specific antibodies with sufficient specificity and in sufficient amounts suitable for _in vivo_ therapy.

Monoclonal antibodies have created a new wave of enthusiasm for using antibodies for the treatment of cancer. Monoclonal antibodies are specific for a single target antigen, can be produced in large quantities with good purity, and can be uniformly coupled to drugs, toxins, and radionuclides. The specificity of monoclonal antibodies should theoretically reduce toxicity to normal tissues that are nonreactive with the antibody conjugate. Unlike crude heteroantisera, the monoclonal antibodies require no absorption, and are of a single immunoglobulin subclass. Monoclonal antibodies can be produced in large quantities from ascites fluid or by tissue culture production techniques and theoretically antibody can be produced indefinitely from hybridomas.

In this book, we review the current status of monoclonal antibody therapy of human cancer. Clinical trials with monoclonal antibodies are being vigorously pursued. Treatment of patients by infusion of unlabeled antibodies has been reported for leukemia, lymphoma, and solid tumors. Recent reports of purging bone marrow with monoclonal antibodies and complement for autologous bone marrow transplantation in leukemia and lymphoma patients offer an exciting alternative approach. Conjugating antibodies to ^{111}indium, ^{131}iodine, and ^{125}iodine for imaging tumors has demonstrated that these conjugates may in some cases detect tumors that could not be identified by standard methods. Imaging trials are the natural predecessors of therapeutic trials with antibodies conjugated to other radionuclides that emit short path length cytotoxic radiation.

In animal models, conjugates of antibody to drugs and toxins have clearly shown their superior cytotoxic effect over unconjugated antibodies.

We anticipate major advances in the treatment of certain types of cancer and are hopeful that the era of the "magic bullet" aptly described by Ehrlich is close at hand.

MONOCLONAL ANTIBODY THERAPY
OF HUMAN CANCER

1. MONOCLONAL ANTIBODY THERAPY OF CANCER: PARAMETERS WHICH AFFECT THE EFFICACY OF IMMUNOTOXINS

ALTON C. MORGAN, JR., ROBERT W. SCHROFF, KOU M. HWANG and GOWSALA PAVANASASIVAM

1. INTRODUCTION

The major problems with the current modalities of cancer therapy are the lack of tumor specificity and the low therapeutic/toxic ratio of anticancer drugs and radiation therapy. A major advance in the treatment of cancer could be heralded by the development of a class of agents that have a greater degree of tumor specificity. The technique of hybridization of an immortal myeloma cell line with an antibody-producing B cell, developed by Köhler and Milstein (1), provides a technique by which monoclonal antibodies with considerable tumor specificity could be produced in unlimited quantities.

Clinical trials evaluating the efficacy, toxicity, pharmacokinetics, and immunogenicity of murine antibodies in humans are currently underway. The use of animal tumor models is also very important in attempting to assess the use of monoclonal antibodies in vivo and, particularly, to assess immunoconjugates in cancer therapeutics. Unconjugated antibodies may be useful against cancer cells through the complement system or by cell-mediated effector functions, but the use of antibody conjugated to drugs, toxins, or radioisotopes offers the greatest hope for the development of cancer-selective cytotoxic reagents.

Conjugates of monoclonal antibody to drugs, toxins, and radioisotopes are currently being tested. Each of these reagents carries its own therapeutic capabilities as well as its own intrinsic toxicities. However, each has the potential for enhanced therapeutic specificity depending on the inherent specificity of the antibody for tumor cells. Because many problems

K.A. Foon and A.C. Morgan, Jr. (eds.), *Monoclonal Antibody Therapy of Human Cancer.* Copyright © 1985. Martinus Nijhoff Publishing, Boston. All rights reserved.

remain to be defined, including the optimal class of immuno-globulin for therapy, the best methods of purification of anti-body, the optimal route and schedule of administration, the immune reactions to the mouse immunoglobulin, and the role of immunoconjugates, this is a fertile field for laboratory and clinical investigation of cancer-selective agents.

In order to assess the numerous variables associated with optimizing monoclonal antibody therapy, conjugates have been examined both in in vitro cell culture systems and to a lesser degree in animal models, primarily murine. For the most part, in vivo animal model results have not proven as impressive as in vitro results would have predicted (2). Nevertheless, the unique capability of MoAb for targeting toxic agents has much potential for the field of cancer therapy. In this chapter, we will address a number of parameters that affect the utility of monoclonal antibodies as carriers of toxins.

2. IN VITRO EVALUATION

2.1. Molecular nature of target antigens

A variety of cell surface targets on tumor cells have been exploited for MoAb toxin studies. These include hormone recep-tors for epithelial growth factor (EGF) and human chorionic gonadotropin (HCG) (3,4) and transferrin receptors (5). For the most part, tumor-associated antigens in humans have been the targets for most studies, including the protein antigen on colon carcinoma cells recognized by antibody 17-1A (6), carcino-embryonic antigen (CEA) (7), alpha fetoprotein (8), the common acute lymphoblastic leukemia antigen (CALLA) (8), p97 (9), and the 250 Kd glycoprotein/proteoglycan complex in melanoma (10,11). In murine systems, T-cell (12) and B-cell lymphoma systems (13) have been the subject of most immunotoxin investigations. The successful use of toxin conjugates in all these systems indicates that the molecular nature of an antigen does not restrict its use as a target structure. However, other factors, which include antigen density and heterogeneity and the degree of modulation or turnover, could greatly influence the utility of a MoAb-toxin conjugate.

2.2. Antigenic heterogeneity

One of the hallmarks of antibody reactivity, as assessed on tissue sections of patient tumors, is antigenic heterogeneity. With the advent of monoclonal antibodies directed at a single epitope on a single antigen species, antigenic heterogeneity has been recognized as a potential major limitation for successful therapeutic applications (14). There is no doubt that the degree of reactivity of a given monoclonal antibody with a given histologic type of tumor is of unparalleled importance in the design and eventual utility of a monoclonal antibody for therapeutic applications. Several reports in the literature have proposed that "cocktails" of antibodies to different antigens on the same tumor will be required for optimal therapeutic use (15,16). There are a number of conceivable explanations for antigenic heterogeneity apparent on tissue sections of tumors. We have examined a number of these explanations in human melanoma using the antibody 9.2.27 to a 250 Kd glycoprotein/proteoglycan. One explanation for antigenic heterogeneity is simply that genetically stable variants exist in a population of tumor cells which do not synthesize or express a given tumor marker. Evidence for this has been obtained for one melanoma-associated antigen using clones derived from cultured melanoma cells (17). We have similarly analyzed clonal populations of primary melanoma and as yet have not found clones lacking the 250 Kd glycoprotein/ proteoglycan complex. However, variants can be sorted by flow cytometry which are stable over long periods in culture for high or low expression of the 250 Kd glycoprotein/proteoglycan, a previously unrecognized phenomenon (18). Second, the state of differentiation of a tumor cell population may influence expression of a given marker. Evidence for this has been found in expression of CEA in colon cancer where more differentiated tumors are more likely to express this marker (19). We have seen no evidence for this with the 250 Kd glycoprotein/proteoglycan. Other laboratories have already reported that the 250 Kd glycoprotein/proteoglycan is present on both primary and metastatic tumors as well as benign nevi (14,20). A third explanation for antigen heterogeneity could be that antigen expression during different phases of the cell cycle is variable. Again, evidence for this has been found with both tumor markers and histocompatibility antigens on human melanoma (21,22). We have found little difference in antigen expression according to the stage of the cell cycle, although there is a higher content of the 250 Kd glycoprotein/proteoglycan on larger cells in G0/G1 phases (23). A fourth explanation for antigenic heterogeneity, as assessed on tissue sections, is one that may be peculiar for the 250 Kd glycoprotein/proteoglycan. We have found that areas of tumor necrosis are often not stained by 9.2.27 antibodies with the indirect immunoperoxidase technique. Possibly in areas of tumor cell lysis, protease levels are increased, leading to antigen fragmentation and loss of epitope for the monoclonal antibody. To this regard, we had previously shown that the 250 Kd glycoprotein/proteoglycan was highly trypsin sensitive (24).

Lastly, antigen heterogeneity could be related to the epitope on an antigen recognized by antibody. Our data have indicated that multiple epitopes exist on the 250 Kd glycoprotein/proteoglycan as recognized by monoclonal antibodies and that all of the epitopes are not found on all 250 Kd glycoprotein/proteoglycan molecules. Our present knowledge indicates that the 9.2.27 antibody recognizes an epitope present on most 250 Kd glycoprotein/proteoglycan molecules whereas other monoclonal antibodies recognize a subset of the molecules recognized by 9.2.27. Recognition of distinct epitopes has important implications for the degree of reactivity of an antibody (Fig. 1). Three antibodies to distinct epitopes were tested by flow cytometry for binding to cultured melanoma cells. The highest reactivity was found with 9.2.27. The same hierarchy of reactivity was found with tissue sections of fresh human melanoma. These distinctions in reactivity on cells and tissue sections correlated with the degree of reactivity to the 250 Kd glycoprotein in gels (Fig. 2). If this phenomenon is shown to have application to other tumor-associated antigens, then not only the analysis of an antigen but also the epitope recognized by an antibody may be important for optimal selection of antibodies for clinical application. This molecular phenomenon has important

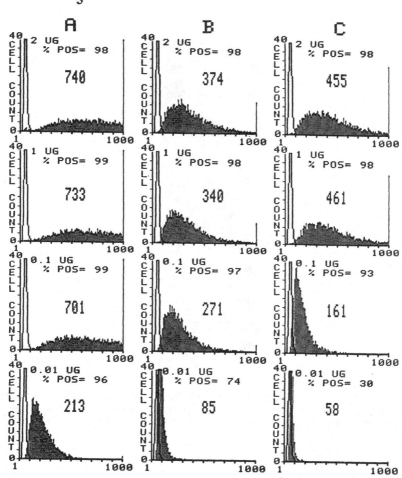

FIGURE 1. Flow cytometry comparison of antibodies to the 250 Kd glycoprotein/proteoglycan. (A) 9.2.27. (B) PG-2. (C) ZME018. Mean fluorescence intensity for each antibody dilution is indicated in the histogram.

implications for antigenic heterogeneity; those antibodies recognizing the smallest subset of molecules have reduced cell surface reactivity as measured by flow cytometry and are more focal and less intense in staining of tissue sections. A similar finding of molecular subsets defined by monoclonal antibodies

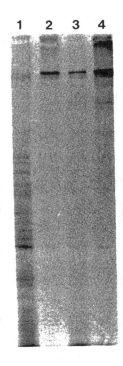

FIGURE 2. Indirect immunoprecipitation and SDS-PAGE comparison of antibodies to the 250 Kd glycoprotein/proteoglycan (lane 1) control myeloma protein (RPC-5). Lane 2: ZME018. Lane 3: PG-2. Lane 4: 9.2.27.

has been recently demonstrated with HLA-DR, where certain subsets of molecules were shown to bear distinct allospecificities (25,26). This phenomenon has also been found with carcinoembryonic antigen where normal cross-reactive antigen (NCA) determinants are found on CEA molecules (27). It has also been well recognized that monoclonal antibodies react with only a portion of labeled CEA molecules that react with polyclonal anti-CEA (25,29).

2.3. Antigenic modulation and internalization

Antigen modulation may be of clinical importance due to the capacity of some tumors to evade the potential effectiveness of unconjugated monoclonal antibody therapy by modulation of the target antigen (30,33). On the other hand, since antigen modulation is often accompanied by internalization of antigen-antibody complexes, as has been demonstrated for the T101 antibody (30) and by Pesando et al. for the J5 antibody to the common acute lymphoblastic leukemia antigen (CALLA) (18), modulation may serve as an efficient means of delivering toxins in the form of immunoconjugates into tumor cells for therapeutic purposes.

We had previously found that the addition of monocytes results in enhanced modulation of the T65 antigen on normal or leukemic lymphoid cells cultured in vitro with the T101 monoclonal antibody (34) (Fig. 3). As shown by the flow cytometry assessment, the decrease in T-65 antigen expression in the presence of monoclonal antibody T101 was enhanced by the addition of monocytes. We extended these findings to demonstrate that monocyte-enhanced modulation is a phenomenon that occurs with a variety of T- and B-lymphoid antigens identified by murine monoclonal antibodies. Two patterns of monocyte-enhanced modulation were observed: 1) augmentation by monocytes of existing antigen modulation, i.e., T101 and anti-Leu-4 antibodies and 2) induction by monocytes of previously unrecognized modulation, i.e., anti-Leu-2 and anti-Leu-9 antibodies. Enhancement of modulation by monocytes was also detected with antibodies to surface IgM and HLA-DR antigens. Monocyte-enhanced modulation is dependent upon the Fc portion of the antibody but independent of proteolytic or oxidative compounds released by monocytes. In vitro studies of antigen modulation were shown to vary with the source of cells and the percent of monocytic cells.

The receptor-mediated endocytosis of a variety of ligands, including antibodies, is believed to be mediated by internalization through coated pits (35,37). The efficiency of internalization varies greatly with different ligands; however, the reason for this variation is not well understood. The enhancing function of monocytes upon antigen modulation may be mediated

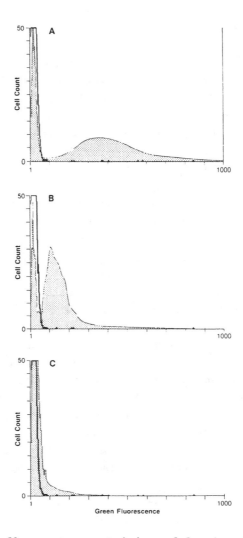

FIGURE 3. Immunofluorescence staining of lymphocyte suspensions modulated with T101 in the presence or absence of monocytes. Histograms represent fluorescence intensity vs. cell number for modulated and unmodulated elutriation-purified lymphocyte suspensions. Lymphocytes were cultured for 3 hr at 37°C in the absence of T101 (A) or with 0.1 µg/ml T101 in the absence (B) or presence (C) of 30% allogeneic monocytes. The fluorescence staining profile of cells incubated in the absence of T101 and stained with RPC-5 as negative controls is included as an open curve in each histogram as a point of reference. Monocytes were gated out of fluorescence analysis.

through aggregation or patching of antibody cell surface antigen complexes on target cells. Although some monocyte Fc receptors might be expected to be occupied by endogenously bound immunoglobulin, immune-complexed antibodies on the lymphoid cell surface could presumably displace the bound human immunoglobulin, allowing patching of antibody-antigen complexes within the target cell surface membrane and/or lateral movement of Fc receptors within the monocyte/macrophage surface membrane. Potentially, these patches of antigen-antibody complexes could then be internalized more rapidly or efficiently than antigen-antibody complexes not cross-linked by monocyte Fc receptors. Conjugates being mixtures of different ratios of antibody and toxins might have variable reactivity with monocyte Fc receptors. Potentially internalization might be increased with multivalent antibody conjugate species. The ability to enhance antigen modulation may be of great importance to the therapeutic use of monoclonal antibody toxin conjugates. Monocyte-mediated enhancement of antigen modulation may serve to augment intracellular uptake of immunoconjugate and optimize the effectiveness of this form of therapy.

We have also examined antigen modulation in two solid tumor systems and examined the role of modulation on the toxicity of conjugates. In these sytems there was no correlation of modulation with the degree of conjugate cytotoxicity. The most striking example was with gelonin and ricin A chain conjugated to the antimelanoma antibody 9.2.27. Neither of these conjugates shows detectable modulation of cell surface antigen, yet they kill antigen-positive melanoma cells at 10^{-11} to 10^{-13} M (ID_{50}). While not showing modulation, the conjugates very rapidly internalized (Fig. 4). Internalization, as measured by loss of trypsin sensitivity of cell-bound antibody, was analyzed on cultured melanoma cells. In contrast to unconjugated 9.2.27, both ricin/A and gelonin conjugates were internalized to a high degree. Thus, internalization was enhanced by conjugation with toxin but yet without detectable modulation. In this case and in other examples of antibodies to antigens on solid tumors and in contrast to lymphoid targets, antigen mobility and internalization may not result in sufficient antigen aggregation to be detected as modulation.

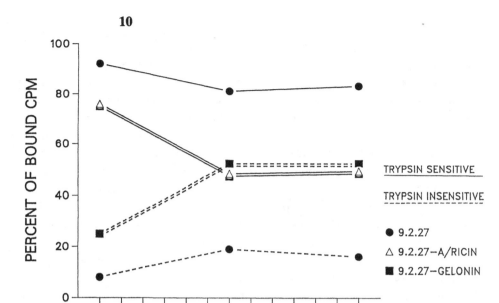

FIGURE 4. Internalization of unconjugated and toxin-conjugated 9.2.27. Antigen-positive melanoma cells were treated with ^{125}I-9.2.27 (●), 9.2.27-ricin/A-^{125} (△), and 9.2.27-gelonin-^{125}I (■) for 1 hr at 4°C, washed, and incubated at 37°C for the indicated periods. At each time point, aliquots of cells were removed, treated with trypsin to remove cell surface bound antibody or conjugate, and the fractions counted. Trypsin-sensitive = cell surface − (————); typsin-insensitive = internal − (− − −).

1.4. Conjugate potency and selectivity

Potency and selectivity in killing antigen-positive cells have been the most intensely studied aspects of toxin conjugates in vitro. Toxin conjugates have been reported to vary in potency from 10^{-7} to 10^{-12} M (ID_{50}) (38,39). The most potent of these toxin conjugates have employed intact ricin (39) or abrin (40) rather than isolated A subunits, resulting in an increase in potency of 100- to 1000-fold. Intact toxins bind to cell surface carbohydrate through a site on the B chain, are internalized presumably through coated pits, and are released into the cytoplasm where the A chain binds to and inactivates the 60S subunit of ribosomes (reviewed by Olsnes and Pihl, ref. 41). Selectivity of intact toxin conjugates has been achieved through either incubation with galactose to inhibit B-chain binding to cell surface carbohydrate (42), covalent incorporation of galactose into the B chain (43), or binding of intact toxin to antibody in such a manner that the carbohydrate binding site of the B chain is sterically occluded (39). The latter technique has shown great promise for increasing the rate of internalization and, thus, the potency of the conjugate. However, a drawback to this procedure can be that a portion of the B chains incorporated into conjugate may still be capable of binding galactose residues and thus removal by affinity chromatography on insolubilized sugar residues is required. The percent of conjugate with exposed B chains is dependent on the type of toxin, as studied with ricin or abrin (40) and, in our hands, the antibody used for conjugation. A second potential drawback of whole toxin conjugates could be release of toxin from conjugate in vivo, leading to toxicity. Thus far, in our experience administration of intact abrin conjugates to guinea pigs and nude mice had little evident toxicity, indicating little release of whole toxin.

A major factor in conjugate potency and selectivity, which has not been well studied, is the antibody-antigen system used for conjugation. We have examined ricin/A and abrin/A, pokeweed antiviral protein (PAP) and gelonin, and whole abrin conjugates of 9.2.27 antibody to human melanoma and D3 antibody to guinea pig L10 hepatocellular carcinoma. All 9.2.27 conjugates were potent (10^{-14} M to 10^{-11} M ID_{50}) and highly selective. D3 antibody, however, formed potent conjugate only with intact abrin but not with any of the A chains or A chain-like toxins (PAP and gelonin). As an example, both D3 and 9.2.27 were conjugated to the same preparation of ricin/A (Fig. 5). Although both conjugates were selective in killing antigen-positive cells, the potencies of the two conjugates are distinctly different. 9.2.27-ricin/A conjugate was 6,000-fold more potent than D3-ricin/A against appropriate antigen-positive cells (5.5 x 10^{-13} M) vs. 3.3 x 10^{-9} M ID_{50}). Our preliminary indication is that the potency of both sets of antibody conjugates correlates with the degree of internalization; 9.2.27 conjugates internalize up to

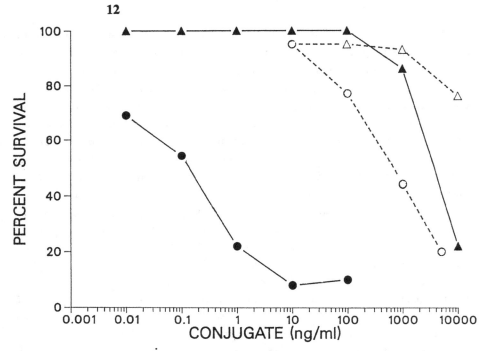

FIGURE 5. Potency and selectivity of two different immunotoxins. Percent survival was measured by ^{3}H-thymidine uptake. (○) D3-ricin/A vs. antigen-positive Ll0 hepatoma cells. (△) D3-ricin/A vs. antigen-negative Ll hepatoma cells. (●) 9.2.27-ricin/A vs. antigen-positive FMX human melanoma cells. (▲) 9.2.27-ricin/A vs. antigen-negative A375 human melanoma cells.

50% in 6 hr, whereas only 10% of the D3-ricin A/chain conjugates internalize over the same interval. Thus, both the type of toxin and the antibody used for conjugation are important in producing potent and selective conjugates.

3. IN VIVO EVALUATION

The properties of conjugates studied in vitro have their corollary in in vivo stuies. In addition, there are several distinct questions that can only be addressed in in vivo animal models.

3.1. Conjugate delivery

The question of delivery or localization to tumor has been primarily addressed with radiolabeled antibodies. However, the results with radiolabeled antibodies may not adequately predict the behavior of radiolabeled toxin conjugates. Preliminary studies have only been recently reported on the biodistribution of a drug conjugate (44). This area is under investigation in a number of laboratories. With this proviso, radiolabeled antibody studies have demonstrated that only a relatively small proportion of the total administered antibody actually localizes to the tumor.

Most antibody administered by the intravenous route remains in the circulation or is distributed in the reticuloendothelial system (RES) organs--lung, liver, and spleen (reviewed by Goldenberg, ref. 45). We have compared murine monoclonal antibody localization and biodistribution in nude mice and in a heterologous species, guinea pigs. The pattern of biodistribution of the same antibody was significantly different in the two species. RES organ and kidney accumulation, two murine monoclonals, was dramatically increased in the heterologous species compared to the homologous species, nude mice. This nonspecific uptake in guinea pigs increased with increasing doses of labeled antibody. These distinctions, if not due to individual species differences, may reflect a host response to homologous vs. heterologous antibody and may be a major problem in clinical application of murine monoclonals. Decreased uptake into the RES organs has been achieved by using intralymphatic administration (46) or by using immunoglobulin fragments.

F(ab')$_2$ fragments seem to be the most generally useful type of fragment because they retain bivalent binding, which has been shown to be important in internalization of toxin conjugate (8), and, with most antibodies, show little loss of affinity, a common problem with monovalent Fab fragments (47). F(ab')$_2$ fragments, however, may have decreased stability in conjugate form or may be susceptible to loss of immunoreactivity in labeled form.

Besides biodistribution, the fate of antibody once bound to tumor cells is an important parameter for immunoconjugate studies. In contrast to antigens like CALLA (8) and T65 (30), which are antigens on lymphoid malignancies which undergo rapid modulation when bound by antibody, many antigens of solid tumors show little modulation (48), as previously discussed. Even though there is not detectable modulation, there can be distinctions in the rate of in vivo turnover. Striking examples of this are the two solid tumor systems we have studied: L10 hepatocellular carcinoma in guinea pigs and human melanoma xenografted in nude mice (Fig. 6). The D3 antibody in L10 tumors shows a rapid accretion into tumor, with a maximum at 24 hr, with an equally rapid loss from tumor, similar to the rate of loss from normal organs. In contrast, the 9.2.27 antibody shows a slower rate of accretion in human melanoma, a steady-state period for up to 5 days, then a gradual loss. These properties affect the quality of tumor imaging (9.2.27, panel A; irrelevant antibody, panel B; D3, panel C; irrelevant antibody, panel D). The localization and turnover of antibody may also affect radiotherapy with α- or β-emitting isotope conjugates, but may have little effect on the efficacy of toxin conjugates. Both antibodies, conjugated to toxins, have shown therapeutic effects against established palpable tumors (11,49).

Low antigen density has not been thought to be a limitation for toxin conjugate therapy. However, for other types of conjugates with drug and therapeutic isotopes, high antigen density should enhance localization and, thus, efficacy. Several monoclonal antibodies recognizing low-density antigens have produced excellent cytotoxic conjugates with toxins, the best example being the J5 antibody to the CALLA antigen (8). Ricin/A-chain conjugated antibody, directed to the p97 antigen on melanoma cells, was shown to kill more efficiently the higher the antigen density (9). This latter finding was also true in vitro with toxin conjugates of antimelanoma antibody 9.2.27. Thus, there is probably a minimal number of cell surface molecules necessary for optimal expression of conjugate toxicity for cultured cells. When this critical density is exceeded, little difference in

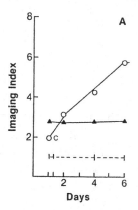

111In 9.2.27/Human Melanoma Xenograft

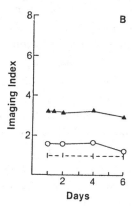

111In D₃/Human Melanoma Xenograft

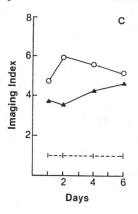

111In D₃/L-10 Hepatoma in Guinea Pig

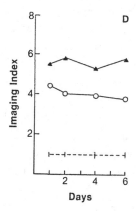

111In 9.2.27/L-10 Hepatocarcinoma in Guinea Pig

FIGURE 6. Variation of imaging index of tumor and major organs as a function of time in two antigen-antibody systems. (A) 111In-9.2.27/human melanoma xenografts in nude mice. (B) 111In-D3/human melanoma xenografts in nude mice. (C) 111In-D3/L10 hepatocarcinoma in guinea pig. (D) 111In-9.2.27/L10 hepatocarcinoma in guinea pig. Imaging indices are presented for tumor (O——O), major organs (▲——▲), and muscle (|---|). Imaging indices were defined by the ratio of specific cpm of tissue to specific cpm of muscle (as background).

potency will be seen with further increase in antigen density. However, a more important question concerns the effect of antigen density on conjugate potency in vivo. There is yet no answer; however, data from our own radiolabeled antibody studies with antimelanoma antibody 9.2.27 indicate that antibody localization is dependent on antigen density. In a nude mouse-human melanoma xenograft system, mice with tumors varying in size from 60 to 4000 mg were injected with nonsaturating levels of labeled antibody (50) (Fig. 7). Comparing tumors of different antigen density, as assessed by flow cytometry, both the percent of the input dose adsorbed into the tumor and the specific activity (cpm/gram tumor tissue) were higher in the high antigen density tumor (SESX) compared with the intermediate antigen-expressing tumor (FMX). In addition, although the total adsorbed dose increased with tumor volume, the specific activity of labeled antibody in the tumor decreased (Fig. 8). These results indicate that the degree of antigen expression in vivo is an important parameter for localization and potentially for the toxic effect of immunoconjugates.

Another factor that could affect localization, and thus therapeutic efficacy, is an immune response to either the antibody or toxin portion of a conjugate. In contrast to earlier clinical trials, primarily with murine monoclonals to lymphoid malignancies, high-dose serotherapy with murine monoclonals in melanoma and colorectal cancer has elicited minimal antiglobulin responses (51-54). A recent report has shown that in mice treated with Thy 1.1 antibody-ricin A and pokeweed antiviral protein (PAP) conjugates, antitoxin antibodies to ricin A or PAP were elicited following a course of conjugate therapy. These antibodies in vitro could neutralize the activity of the conjugate (55). The same report showed that the neutralizing antibodies to ricin A did not cross-react with antibodies to PAP, suggesting that alternating courses of immunoconjugates with different toxin polypeptides could avoid the detrimental effect of the host immune response. Other solutions might include a variety of tolerization methods, including antigen-induced B-cell suicide in which either the antigen or anti-idiotypic antibody

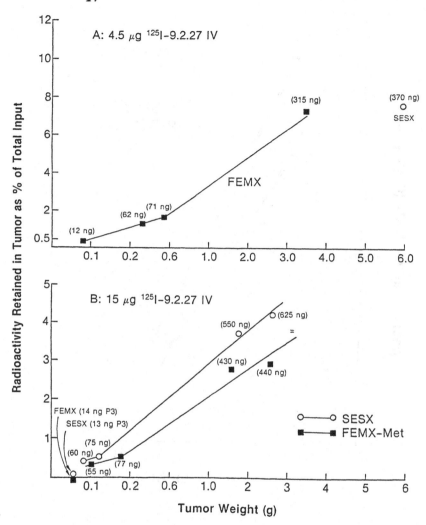

FIGURE 7. Uptake of ^{125}I-9.2.27 by human melanoma xenografts of various sizes. (A) BALB/c nude mice bearing different sizes of FMX-Met were injected with 4.5 µg ^{125}I-9.2.27 (3 µCi/µg). The animals were sacrificed and tumor removed 54 hr after injection. The radiaoctivity was determined by γ-scintillation counter. (B) BALB/c nude mice bearing human melanoma xenografts (SESX, FMX) were injected with either 15 µg ^{125}I-9.2.27 (5 µCi/µg). Fifty-four hours later the animals were sacrificed and the radioactivity accumulated in the tumor was determined by γ-scintillation counter.

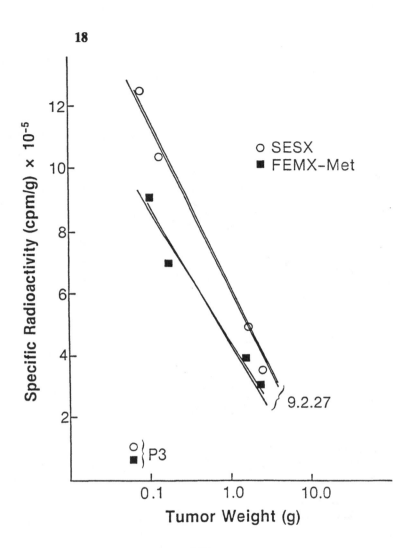

FIGURE 8. Specific uptake of [125]I-9.2.27 as a function of tumor burden. The experiment was performed as described above.

could be conjugated to toxin and targeted to B cells responding to the conjugate or the use of less immunogenic toxin polypeptides for conjugation, as has been claimed with α-amanitin (37). Regardless, future clinical trials with conjugates must monitor host immune response to both antibody and toxin components of conjugate.

3.2. Tumor burden

For evaluation of therapeutic efficacy of toxin, drug, and radiotherapeutic conjugates, investigations have utilized, for the most part, animal models in which the tumor burden has been limited and the tumors not established (2,12,43). When tumor burden has been increased or the therapeutic regimen delayed until several days after injection of the tumor inoculum, the effect of conjugates on tumor growth has been minimal (2). The lack of success of conjugates against larger tumor burdens may be due to any of the previous questions that have been addressed thus far, including in vivo turnover and antigenic heterogeneity, but may also be due to administration of insufficient conjugate. Based on in vitro potency, small doses of conjugate should be sufficient. However, based on our own studies with trace-labeled 9.2.27, gelonin conjugates localized 8-fold less and ricin conjugates 15-fold less well than unconjugated antibody. The decreased localization can be accounted for by the greatly shortened serum half-life of conjugates which have a T 1/2 of 6 hr vs. 36 hr with unconjugated antibody. Thus, approximately 0.01% or less of the conjugate dose reaches the tumor site in a small, palpable tumor. For larger tumors, it would be expected that even fewer antibody molecules localize per cell. Thus, a potential solution to dealing with increased tumor burden is to increase the amount of conjugate injected, assuming that toxicity would not be limiting, or to increase tumor localization by inhibiting non-antigen-specific uptake. A third attractive alternative is to utilize models in which therapy can be directed at established microscopic metastases to which conjugated might be more effectively targeted. We have, therefore, treated guinea pigs with primary tumors and microscopic lymph node disease with abrin-A-chain conjugate and found we could inhibit the onset and subsequent growth of the lymph node metastasis (49).

Another approach that has already been successfully used is combining immunconjugate therapy with "debulking" therapies like radiation or chemotherapy. Employed in a murine chronic lympho-cytic leukemia model, the combination of radiation, splenectomy, and conjugate therapy resulted in cures (56). This approach could be further extrapolated to the use of combinations of immunoconjugates or to combining different toxic agents within the same conjugate. The latter approach could conceivably combine agents, such as intact ricin or abrin, which internalize well, with drugs which may not internalize well. It is hoped that future *in vivo* animal model studies will identify new combinations of agents which act in a synergistic fashion and that the efficacy of these combinations of agents can be enhanced by conjugation to specific antibody.

REFERENCES

1. Köhler G, Milstein C. 1975. Nature (London) 256:495-797.
2. Blythman HE, Casellas P, Gros O, et al. 1981. Nature 290: 145-146.
3. Oeltman TN, Heath EC. 1979. J Biol Chem 254:1028-1031.
4. Cawley DB, Herschman HR, Gilliland DG, Collier RJ. 1980 Cell 22:563-570.
5. Trowbridge IS, Domingo DL. 1981. Nature 294:171-173.
6. Gilliland DG, Steplewski Z, Collier RJ, Mitchell RF, Chang TH, Koprowski H. 1980. Proc Natl Acad Sci USA 77:4539.
7. Levin LV, Griffin TW, Haynes LR, Sedor CJ. 1982. J Biol Resp Modif 1:149-162.
8. Raso V, Ritz J, Basala M, Schlossman S. 1982. Cancer Res 42:457-464.
9. Casellas P, Brown JP, Gros O, et al. 1982. Int J Cancer 30:437-444.
10. Bumol TF, Wang QC, Reisfeld RA, Kaplan NO. 1983. Proc Natl Acad Sci USA 80:529-533.
11. Morgan AC Jr, Pavanasasivam G, Hwang KM, et al. 1984. In: Protides of the Biological Fluids (Ed H Peeters), Elsevier, Amsterdam, in press.
12. Houston LL, Nowinski RC. 1981. Cancer Res 41:3913-3917.
13. Krolick KA, Villemez C, Isakson P, Uhr JW, Vitteta ES. 1980. Proc Natl Acad Sci USA 77:5419-5423.
14. Albino AP, Lloyd KO, Houghton AN, Oettgen HF, Old LJ. 1981. J Exp Med 154:1764-1778.
15. Natali PG, Cavaliere R, Bigotti A, et al. J Immunol 130: 1462-1466.
16. Marx JL. 1981. Science 216:283-285.
17. Yeh M-Y, Hellström I, Hellström KE. 1981. J Immunol 126:1312-1317.
18. Lindmo R, Davies C, Fodstad Ø, Morgan AC Jr. 1985. Int J Cancer, in press.
19. Nakapoulou L, Zinozi M, Theodoropoulos G, Papacharalampous N. 1982. Dis Colon Rectum 26:269-274.
20. Hellström I, Carrigues HJ, Cabasco L, Mosely GH, Brown JP, Hellström KE. 1983. J Immunol 130:1467-1472.
21. Burshiel SW, Martin JC, Imai K, Ferrone S, Warner NL. 1982. Cancer Res 42:4110-4115.

22. Sarkan S, Glassy MC, Ferrone S, Jones OW. 1980. Proc Natl Acad Sci USA 77:7297-7301.
23. Lindmo T, Davies C, Rotstad EK, Fodstad Ø, Sundan A. 1984. Int J Cancer, in press.
24. Morgan AC Jr, Galloway DR, Reisfeld RA. 1981. Hybridoma 1: 27-36.
25. Quaranta V, Pellegrino MA, Ferrone S. 1981. J Immunol 126:548-552.
26. Quaranta V, Tanigaki N, Ferrone S. 1981. Immunogenetics 12:175-182.
27. Primus FJ, Kuhns WJ, Goldenberg DM. 1983. Cancer Res 43: 693-701.
28. Primus RJ, Newell KD, Blue A, Goldenberg DM. 1983. Cancer Res 43:686-692.
29. Rogers GT, Rowlins GA, Keep PA, Cooper EH, Bagshawe KD. 1981. Br J Cancer 44:371-380.
30. Schroff RW, Farrell MM, Klein RA, Oldham RK, Foon KA. 1985. J Immunol, in press.
31. Foon KA, Schroff RW, Bunn PA, et al. 1985. Blood, in press.
32. Foon KA, Bunn PA, Schroff RW, et al. In: Monoclonal Antibodies and Cancer (Eds BD Boss, RE Langman, I Trowbridge, R Dulbecco), Academic Press, New York, p 39.
33. Ritz J, Pesando JM, Sallan SE, et al. 1981. Blood 58:141.
34. Schroff RW, Klein RA, Farrell MM, Stevenson HC. 1984. J Immunol 133:1641.
35. Pastan I, Willingham MC. 1983. Trends Biochem Sci 8:250.
36. Steinman RM, Mellman IS, Muller WA, Cohn ZA. 1983. J Cell Biol 96:1.
37. Unkeless JC, Fleit H, Mellman IS. 1981. Adv Immunol 31:247.
38. David M-TB, Preston JF. 1981. Science 213:1385-1387.
39. Thorpe PE, Ross WC, Brown AN, et al. 1984. Eur J Biochem 140:63-71.
40. Godal A, Funderud S, Fodstad Ø, Pihl A. 1984. In: Protides of the Biological Fluids (Ed H Peeters), Elsevier, Amsterdam, in press.
41. Olsnes S, Pihl A. 1982. In: Molecular Actions of Toxins and Viruses (Eds PL Cohen, S van Heyningen), Elsevier, Amsterdam.
42. Vallera DA, Youle RJ, Neville DM, Kersey JH. 1982. J Exp Med 155:949.
43. Houston LL. 1983. J Biol Chem 258:7208-7212.
44. Vadia P, Blair AH, Ghose T. 1984. Cancer Res 44:4263-4266.
45. Goldenberg DM. 1983. J Nucl Med 24:360-362.
46. Weinstein JN, Steller MA, Keenan AM, et al. 1983. Science 222:423-426.
47. Wahl RL, Parker CW. Philpott GW. 1983. J Nucl Med 24:316-325.
48. Hellström I, Brown JP, Hellström KE. 1983. Int J Cancer 31:553-556.
49. Hwang KM, Foon KA, Cheung PH, Pearson JW, Oldham RK. 1984. Cancer Res, in press.
50. Hwang KM, Morgan AC Jr, Fodstad Ø, Oldham RK. 1984. Cancer Res, in press.
51. Oldham RK, Foon KA, Morgan AC, et al. 1984. J Clin Oncol, in press.
52. Schroff RW, Foon KA, Beatty SM, Oldham RK, Morgan AC Jr. 1984. Cancer Res, in press.

53. Sears HF, Mattis J, Herlyn D, et al. 1982. Lancet 1:762-765.
54. Sears HF, Herlyn D, Steplewski Z, Koprowski H. 1984. J Biol Resp Modif 3:138-150.
55. Ramakrishnan S, Houston LL. 1984. Cancer Res 44:1398-1404.
56. Krolick KA, Uhr JW, Slavin S, Vitteta ES. 1982. J Exp Med 155:1797-1809.

2. DESIGN AND DEVELOPMENT OF DRUG-MONOCLONAL ANTIBODY 791T/36 CONJUGATE FOR CANCER THERAPY*

R.W. BALDWIN

1. INTRODUCTION

A fundamental objective in cancer therapy is to destroy malignant cells while minimizing damage to normal cells and tissues.
To this end there is renewed interest in antibody targeting of
antitumor agents including chemotherapeutic drugs, plant and
bacterial toxins, and biological response modifying agents
(1-5).

The choice of an agent for antibody targeting will be influ-
enced by the specificity of the antibody. Theoretically it is
most desirable to target highly toxic agents such as plant
toxins or their A-chain moieties which can kill target cells
following internalization of only a few molecules (4,5). In
this case the antibody vector ideally should be highly specific
for the tumor target cell and readily internalize following
antibody-toxin conjugate binding. In this respect, few if any
of the present murine monoclonal antibodies which react with
human tumors display the specificity which is required for
targeting highly toxic molecules. However, toxin A chain
conjugates have not proved as cytotoxic as was originally
expected (4,5).

An alternative approach is to target cytotoxic drugs which
are already in clinical use and where toxic side effects are
known. There are several pathways which can be exploited for
antibody-directed delivery of drugs (Fig. 1). Drug may be
released following binding of antibody conjugates to antigens
expressed at the tumor cell surface and subsequent internalization (pathway A, Fig. 1). Also, drug moieties may be released

---

*These studies were supported by a grant from the Cancer
Research Campaign.

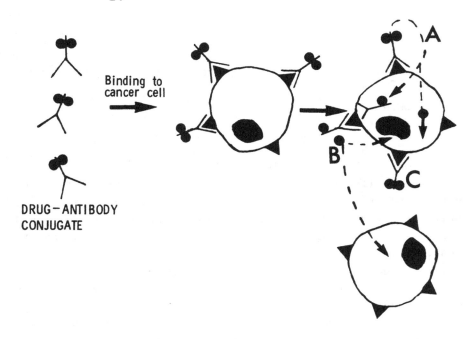

DRUG—ANTIBODY CONJUGATE

Binding to cancer cell

FIGURE 1. Pathways for targeting tumors cytotoxic agents linked to monoclonal antitumor antibodies. Following binding the conjugate may enter the cell intact allowing the drug component to produce its cytotoxic reaction (A). The drug component may be released at the cancer cell surface and then function as free drug (B). Bound complexes may persist at the cell surface (C).

extracellularly by cleavage of drug-antibody bonds following conjugate localization (pathway B). In this case, although it is desirable for the antibody to localize specifically upon tumor cells, antibodies binding to extracellular products such as CEA may be effective; this will considerably increase the potential of antibody targeting systems. Finally, drug-antibody conjugates may be able to inhibit cellular functions, following conjugate binding to tumor cells, even though they remain localized at the tumor cell surface. This pathway has been proposed, for example, with anthracyclines where membrane binding rather than intracellular interactions may account for their cytotoxicity (6).

The design and evaluation of drug-antibody conjugates will be considered principally with respect to the application of a monoclonal antibody designated 791T/36, but the general concepts are applicable to other antibodies to tumor cells. Monoclonal antibody 791T/36 was produced from a hybridoma obtained following fusion of splenocytes from a mouse immunized against cells of a human osteogenic sarcoma (791T) and murine myeloma P3NS1 (7). It was shown to react with 7/14 osteogenic sarcoma cell lines in a radioimmunoassay but did not react with normal fibroblast cultures, several of these fibroblast cultures being derived from donors of positive tumors, including the donor of 791T (7). Primary and metastatic osteogenic sarcomas also react with 791T/36 antibody as demonstrated by immunoperoxidase staining of surgically derived tumor specimens (8). The antibody reacted against some unrelated tumor cell lines, notably colorectal carcinomas (3/5 positive), and with other tumor types reactivity was restricted to isolated examples or not detected at all (7).

The 791T/36 antibody (IgG_{2b} isotype) proved to be stable to labeling with tracers such as radioiodine and fluorescein isothiocyanate (9) and has been estimated to bind to at least 10^6 sites on the surface of 791T cells (10). The epitope has been identified on cultured human osteogenic sarcoma cells as a glycoprotein of apparent molecular weight 72,000 (11). Radioiodinated 791T/36 localized specifically in subcutaneous xenografts of 791T and other antigenically positive tumor lines in immunologically deficient mice when administered intraperitoneally (9) and has also been used successfully in the radioimmunodetection of osteogenic sarcoma and colorectal, breast, and ovarian carcinomas in patients (12-15). These properties established its potential for drug targeting. It fulfills the basic requirements for a high number of antigen-binding sites on appropriate target cells and adequate resistance to inactivation by chemical substitution. The availability of tumor targets with known binding activity both _in vivo_ and _in vitro_ allows for the design of appropriate assays for determining the biological activity of drug-791T/36 conjugates.

2. METHOTREXATE-791T/36 ANTIBODY CONJUGATES

Methotrexate (MTX) was selected as an antineoplastic agent for conjugating to 791T/36 monoclonal antibody in view of its clinical usage, and because it was highly cytotoxic for the 791T osteosarcoma cell line (3,16). This is illustrated in Table 1, which shows the sensitivity of 791T cells to various antineoplastic agents. Tumor cells were incubated for 24 hours with various concentrations of each drug and the tumor cell survival determined using "post-incubation labeling" with ^{75}Se-methionine (^{75}Se-met). From these tests it was established that the most active drugs against tumor 791T were methotrexate, vindesine, and the anthracyclines adriamycin and daunomycin. (IC_{50} 1-5 x 10^{-8} M/ml culture medium.)

2.1. Methotrexate linked directly to 791T/36 antibody

Conjugates were prepared by an activated-ester method using the N-hydroxysuccinimide ester of methotrexate. This was prepared by incubating equimolar quantities of methotrexate, N-hydroxysuccinimide, and dicyclohexyl carbodiimide in a small volume of dimethyl formamide for several hours (16). Substituted 791T/36 antibody was then prepared by reacting the MTX ester with antibody in phosphate-buffered saline. This simple

Table 1. Cytotoxicity of various drugs for 791T human osteogenic sarcoma cell 791T.

	IC_{50}[a] against 791T target cells	
Drug	ng/ml culture medium	Approximate molarity
Methotrexate	5	10^{-8}
Vindesine	10	10^{-8}
Adriamycin	10	2×10^{-8}
Daunomycin	30	5×10^{-8}
Cis-platinum	100	3×10^{-7}
5-fluorouracil	800	5×10^{-7}
5-fluorodoxyuridine	1,400	5×10^{-7}
Melphalan	400	10^{-6}
Retinoic acid	15,000	2×10^{-5}
Interferon	(IC_{50} not reached at 10^5 units/ml)	

[a]Drug concentration inhibiting ^{75}Se-met incorporation by 50%.

and mild chemical reaction made possible the preparation of MTX-791T/36 antibody conjugates (directly linked) with an average molar substitution rate in the range 2.0-3.0. Higher substitution rates invariably resulted in loss of antibody reactivity.

2.2. Methotrexate-HSA-791T/36 antibody conjugate

Directly linked MTX-antibody conjugates were limited by the amount of MTX which could be coupled to antibody, and so conjugates were also prepared using drug carriers. In this approach the molar substitution ratio is limited only by the number of available functional groups for MTX conjugation and the stability and solubility of the substituted carrier under physiological conditions. A wide variety of carriers have been previously investigated for drug delivery but we have utilized human serum albumin (HSA). These conjugates were prepared using a three-step procedure (16). First, MTX-substituted HSA was prepared, while 791T/36 antibody was substituted with iodoacetyl. MTX-HSA-791T/36 antibody conjugates were synthesized by reaction of these two components (Fig. 2).

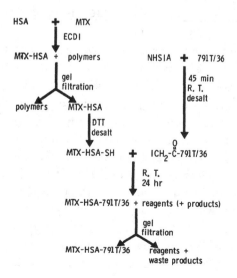

FIGURE 2. Flow diagram of MTX-HSA-791T/36 conjugate synthesis.

In particular, HSA-MTX was synthesized by reacting an excess of methotrexate and ethyl carbodiimide with HSA and unwanted polymerized HSA-methotrexate products were removed by size exclusion chromatography. Iodoacetyl-substituted 791T/36 antibody was produced by reacting a 3- to 4-fold molar excess of N-hydroxy succinimidyl iodoacetate with antibody followed by desalting on a Sephadex G25 column.

HSA-MTX conjugates contain a free sulphydryl group which is in an oxidized unreactive' form. This sulphydryl group was reduced using 50 mM dithiothreitol, and after desalting, was reacted with iodoacetyl-substituted 791T/36 antibody. The reaction products were then separated by size exclusion chromatography as illustrated in Figure 3. This shows the profile of a MTX-HSA 791T/36 antibody conjugate in which the HSA component was trace labeled with ^{125}I-iodine to facilitate component characterization (16). In this particular preparation, the molar ratio of MTX to HSA in the monomeric MTX-HSA was 32:1. Accordingly, the proposed structure of the conjugate (Fig. 4) indicates that each 791T/36 antibody molecule would be able to target 32 MTX residues.

2.3. Characterization of MTX-791T/36 antibody conjugates

2.3.1. Antibody immunoreactivity.

As already indicated, conjugates of antitumor monoclonal antibodies require adequate retention of immunoreactivity. To test this, a flow cytometry technique was developed which measures the capacity of antibody conjugates to compete with fluorescein isothiocyanate-labeled 791T/36 antibody (FITC-791T/36) binding to tumor cells (10). This procedure has several advantages over other tumor cell binding assays such as radioimmunoassays, and in particular allows measurement of antibody binding to cell surface antigens on single cells within homogeneous and heterogeneous populations. It also permits the kinetics of association and dissociation of conjugates to be determined. This is important in establishing the "dwell time" of antibody-targeted agents in the environment of target tumor cells.

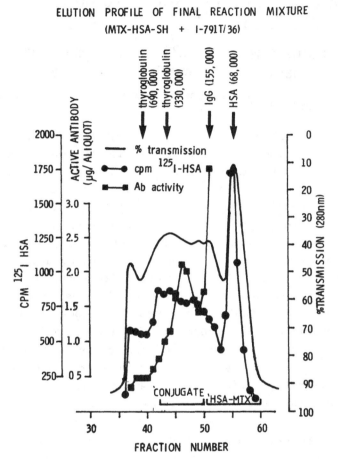

ELUTION PROFILE OF FINAL REACTION MIXTURE
(MTX-HSA-SH + I-791T/36)

FIGURE 3. Elution profile of products from the final reaction mixture assessed by different criteria. Transmittance at 180 nm representing the sum of molecular species present, cpm of ^{125}I representing HSA/MTX content, and antibody activity as measured by flow cytofluorimetry are plotted against fraction number. The sample (3 ml) was eluted from a Fractogel TSK-HW55S column (85 x 2.5 cm) using PBS at a flow rate of 15 mg/hr. Fractions were of 4.2 ml. The thyroglobulin standard contained both whole protein (690 daltons) and subunits (330 daltons).

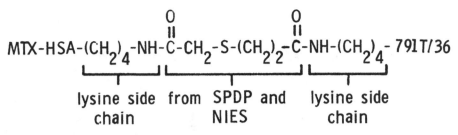

FIGURE 4. Composition of methotrexate human serum albumin-monoclonal antibody 791T/36.

In the competitive inhibition assay, 791T tumor cells are incubated with fluorescein isothiocyanate-labeled 791T/36 antibody (FITX-791T/36) mixed with a range of doses of the competing (unlabeled) antibody, this being either unmodified 791T/36 or antibody conjugate. The degree of inhibition of FITC-791T/36 antibody binding to tumor cells by conjugates is then compared with that obtained with unmodified 791T/36 antibody. These immunofluorescence tests are carried out using a FACS IV flow cytofluorimeter (ref. 10 for technical details). Linear amplification was used to quantitate mean fluorescence intensity, and fluorescence signals were amplified logarithmically for direct comparison of fluorescence intensity. The results are expressed as mean fluorescence intensity per cell which represents the mean fluorescence intensity per cell with FITC-791T/36 antibody-treated tumor cells minus the background mean fluorescence intensity per cell with medium-treated target cells.

As shown in Table 2, the reduction in binding of FITC-791T/36 antibody by unlabeled antibody is very close to the expected reductions. For example, treatment of 791T cells with FITC-791T/36 antibody (1 µg) containing unlabeled 791T/36 antibody (2 µg) would be expected to reduce FITC-791T/36 antibody binding by 66% and the actual measured reduction was 65%. The tests summarized in Table 2 also determined antibody binding to 791T cells by uptake of ^{125}I since the antibody was dual-labeled with FITC and ^{125}I. In agreement with the FACS assays, reduction of ^{125}I-labeled antibody uptake by unlabeled antibody was close to the expected value (10).

Table 2. Inhibition of 791T cell binding of 791T/36 antibody labeled with fluorescein isothiocyanate and ^{125}I by competition with unlabeled 791T/36 antibody.

Unlabeled 791T/36 antibody added to FITC-791T/36[a]	Expected reduction in antibody binding	Fluorescence analysis		Radioisotopic analysis	
		Fluorescence intensity	Percent reduction	Mean cpm bound/ 10^5 cells	Percent reduction
–	–	935	–	1816 ± 7	–
4	80	197	79	435 ± 67	76
2	66	328	65	628 ± 19	65
1	50	493	47	965 ± 61	47
0.5	33	661	29	1157 ± 52	36
0.25	20	771	18	1502 ± 63	17

[a]791T tumor cells incubated with 791T/36 antibody (1 g/2 x 10^5 cells) dual labeled with FITC and ^{125}I with or without added unlabeled 791T/36 antibody for 4 hours. Cells were then washed and all bound ^{125}I and FITC measured (see ref. 10).

Figure 5 illustrates microfluorimetry tests on the inhibition of FITC-791T/36 antibody binding by unmodified 791T/36 antibody and an MTX-conjugate. In this particular conjugate (molar substitution 2.7:1 MTX:antibody) there was a high (75%) retention of antibody reactivity. However, there was considerable loss of antibody reactivity when more than 4 MTX residues were directly linked to antibody. Conjugates prepared using human serum albumin and containing up to 32 moles of MTX/mole antibody retain approximately 30% of the reactivity of unsubstituted antibody (16).

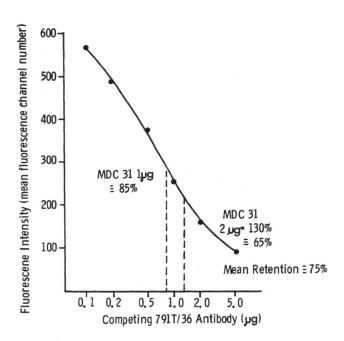

FIGURE 5. Competition of binding of FITC-labeled 791T/36 antibody with 791T cells by unconjugated 791T/36 antibody and a methotrexate conjugate (MDC31) (cf. Table 2 for technique).

2.3.2. <u>In vitro cytotoxicity</u>. The <u>in vitro</u> cytotoxicity of MTX-791T/36 antibody conjugates was measured in a 24-hour assay in which target tumor cells in microtiter plates were cultured with a range of concentrations of conjugate and tumor cell survival estimated by post-labeling with ^{75}Se-met.

Direct MTX-791T/36 antibody conjugates were tested against osteogenic sarcoma 791T cells, which express approximately 10^6 791T/36 antibody-binding sites per cell, and bladder carcinoma T24, which express approximately 10^4 binding sites. The conjugates were cytotoxic for both target tumor cells but with reduced activity compared to that of free MTX (Table 3). Moreover, the 24-hour incubation assay did not demonstrate any discrimination between the cytotoxic effects of MTX-antibody conjugate on 791T and T24 cells. In related trials with other antibody conjugates (see later), specificity of conjugate selectivity has been demonstrated using a "pretreatment assay" in

Table 3. Cytotoxicity of directly linked methotrexate-791T/36 monoclonal antibody conjugates.

| | | Cytotoxicity (IC_{50})[a] against: | |
| | | Osteogenic | Bladder |
Assay	Reagent	sarcoma 791T	carcinoma T24
Chronic assay (24-hr exposure)	MTX	5 ng/ml	2 ng/ml
	MTX-791T/36 (MDC 27)	180 ng/ml	100 ng/ml
	MTX-791T/36 (MDC 30)	180 ng/ml	180 ng/ml
Pretreatment assay (15-min exposure)	MTX	9 µg/ml	8 µg/ml
	MTX-791T/36 (MDC 27) MTX-791T/36 (MDC 30)	nontoxic at 40 µg/ml	nontoxic at 40 µg/ml

[a]Concentration in terms of MTX in culture medium producing 50% inhibition of tumor cell survival as estimated by ^{75}Se-met incorporation.

which tumor cells are incubated with conjugate for 15 minutes, then washed to remove unbound conjugate. Tumor cells are then cultured in microtiter plates for 24 hours and cell survival assessed following ^{75}Se-met labeling (17). But as shown in Table 3, MTX-791T/36 antibody conjugates showed no significant reactivity even against 791T tumor cells, suggesting that these directly linked conjugates are unable to deliver adequate amounts of drug.

Indirect conjugates employing an HSA carrier were more reactive. Table 4 summarizes tests with MTX, MTX-HSA conjugate, and MTX-HSA-791T/36 antibody conjugates, using both the 24-hour and pretreatment assay. MTX-HSA was much less toxic than free MTX for both 791T and T24 target cells. However, the MTX-HSA-791T/36 conjugate was highly cytotoxic for 791T cells. Generally, MTX-HSA-791T/36 conjugates were almost as active as free MTX in terms of MTX concentration but the best preparation had twice the activity of free drug.

Table 4. Cytotoxicity of methotrexate-human serum albumin-791T/36 antibody conjugates.

| Assay | Reagent | Cytotoxicity (IC_{50})[a] against: | |
		Osteogenic sarcoma 791T	Bladder carcinoma T24
Chronic assay (24-hr exposure)	MTX	5 ng/ml	2 ng/ml
	MTX-HSA	900 ng/ml	800 ng/ml
	MTX-HSA-791T/36 Conjugate MT5	18 ng/ml	250 ng/ml
	Conjugate MT17	25 ng/ml	300 ng/ml
Pretreatment assay (15-min exposure)	MTX	9 µg/ml	8 µg/ml
	MTX-HSA	Nontoxic at 40 µg/ml	Nontoxic at 40 µg/ml
	MTX-HSA-791T/36 Conjugate MT5	300 ng/ml	Nontoxic at 40 µg/ml

[a]Concentration in terms of MTX in culture medium producing 50% inhibition of tumor cell survival as estimated by ^{75}Se-met incorporation.

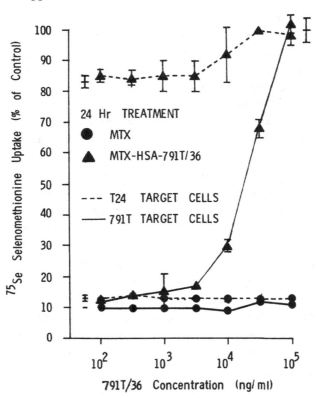

FIGURE 6. The effect of increasing concentrations of free antibody on the cytotoxicity of conjugate and free methotrexate at
100 ng/ml methotrexate concentration against 791T and T24 cells
as targets in a chronic 24-hr cytotoxicity test, measured by the
inhibition of ^{75}Se-met incorporation. Error bars demonstrate the
standard error for each sample and where absent indicate that SE
was less than the plotted point size. The error bar to the right
of the figure demonstrates the error for the medium control. The
error bars to the left of the figure from top to bottom, respectively, show the SE of the conjugate on T24 cells, conjugate on
791T cells and methotrexate on T24 cells, and methotrexate on
791T cells when no competing antibody was present.

The requirement for 791T/36 antibody binding to MTX-HSA-
791T/36 conjugate toxicity was demonstrated by competition
assays, illustrated in Figure 6. In these tests target cells
(osteogenic sarcoma 791T and bladder carcinoma T24) were incubated for 24 hours with either MTX or MTX-HSA-791T/36 in the
presence of increasing amounts of 791T/36 antibody and then

cell survival measured by ^{75}Se-met incorporation. The amount of MTX in free form or in the antibody conjugate in culture medium was 100 ng/ml which previous tests indicated to be the minimum amount giving a maximum cytotoxic response. The cytotoxicity of free MTX for both target cells was not affected by the presence of 791T/36 antibody. However, increasing amounts of antibody reduced the cytotoxic response of MTX-HSA-791T/36 for 791T cells and it was completely abolished in the presence of 10^5 ng/ml.

2.3.3. Clonogenic assay. In vitro cytotoxicity assays, measuring short-term survival of tumor cells synthesis (by incorporation of ^{75}Se-met), may not accurately reflect the cytotoxic potential of MTX or conjugates. Thus, we further assessed conjugates using clonogenic assays in which the long-term growth potential of treated tumor cells was measured. These assays were performed by plating 200 tumor cells in 30-mm culture dishes and incubating for 5-7 days in the continuous presence of MTX or MTX conjugates, after which cell colonies were stained and enumerated. In a typical clonogenic assay (Fig. 7), MTX-HSA-791T/36 antibody conjugate at a dose of approximately 5 ng/ml completely inhibited 791T colony formation and the 50% inhibition dose was 0.3 ng/ml. In comparison, bladder carcinoma T24 cells were much less susceptible to MTX-HSA-791T/36 conjugate although MTX was toxic to both cell lines.

Using the colony inhibition assay it was possible to investigate more closely exposure conditions affecting the action of MTX-HSA-791T/36 conjugates. Table 5 shows experiments in which 791T cells were treated with conjugate at different concentrations, either continuously or discontinuously with alternating culture in growth medium alone. The concentrations chosen were 0.5 ng/ml (IC_{90}) and 10 ng/ml (IC_{100}).

If conjugate exposure was limited to 2 days, followed by a 4-day recovery period, colony formation was approximately 30% greater than in continuously treated cultures at the IC_{90} dose. When cells were allowed to establish small colonies (at 2 days), before exposure to MTX-HSA-791T/36, the conjugate did not completely kill them. The high dose (10 ng/ml) inhibited further

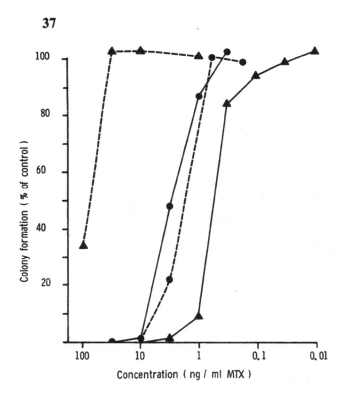

FIGURE 7. Cytotoxicity of MTX-HSA-791T/36 conjugate MT5 against
791T osteogenic sarcoma and T24 bladder carcinoma cells as
measured by colony inhibition assay. Conjugate concentration
is expressed in terms of MTX content and colony formation is
expressed as a percentage of the number of colonies formed in
growth medium controls. ▲----▲ T24 cells treated with conjugate
MT5; ●---● T24 cells treated with MTX; ▲——▲791T cells
treated with conjugate MT5; ●——●791T cells treated with MTX.

cell division so that the mean colony size showed minimal
change, but the IC90 dose allowed colony growth to continue,
albeit at a lower rate and incidence than in controls. These
results show that the conjugate acted in a cytostatic rather
than cytolytic fashion when the target cells were in a logarith-
mic growth phase. Cytostatic inhibition was most effective in
single cells before division had occurred and was a relatively
slow process in that many cells, exposed for 2 days to a partially toxic dose, could still recover in fresh growth medium.
The slow kinetics of cytotoxicity explain the failure of MTX-
HSA-791T/36 to achieve more than about 90% inhibition of

Table 5. Effect of alternating treatment with growth medium and MTX-HSA-791T/36 conjugate on colony formation by 791T cells.

Treatment		Mean no. colonies ± SE	Percent inhibition of colony formation	Mean colony size (No. cells ± SE)
Days 1-2	Days 3-6			
Growth medium[a]	–	142 ± 4[b]	–	4.8 ± 0.3
Growth medium	Growth medium	215 ± 7	0	61.3 ± 11.0
MT5 0.5 ng/ml[c]	MT5 0.5 ng/ml	20 ± 3	91	
MT5 10 ng/ml	MT5 10 ng/ml	0.7 ± 0.2	99.8	
MT5 0.5 ng/ml	Growth medium	76 ± 2	65	
MT5 10 ng/ml	Growth medium	2 ± 1	99	
Growth medium	MT5 0.5 ng/ml	145 ± 3	33	31.8 ± 8
Growth medium	MT5 10 ng/ml	129 ± 7	40	5.9 ± 0.6

[a]These cells were stained after 2 days.
[b]Cultures contained cell pairs which were not scored as colonies.
[c]Expressed as concentration of MTX.

^{75}Se-met uptake over 24 hours at high concentrations. However, when inhibited single cells were forced to remain in the environment of conjugates rather than being allowed to recover, they died within the 5- to 7-day period of the colony inhibition assay, since dishes treated continuously with conjugate contain no single cells at the higher concentration.

2.3.4. Correlation between in vitro cytotoxicity and tumor cell binding of MTX-HSA-791T/36 antibody conjugates. The level of MTX-HSA-791T/36 antibody conjugate binding to 791T tumor cells was measured under conditions used to assay their cytotoxicity in vitro either by inhibition of protein synthesis or colony formation by treated tumor cells. In these tests, 791T cells were incubated with MTX-HSA-791T/36 conjugate using a range of concentrations. Tumor cells were then washed at 4°C and bound MTX-HSA-791T/36 conjugate detected by labeling at 4°C with FITC-labeled rabbit anti-HSA antibody. The fluorescence signal of tumor cells was determined, as already described for FITC-labeled antibody assays, by flow cytometry. These tests, illustrated in Figure 8, indicate that the amount of MTX-HSA-791T conjugate required to deliver sufficient MTX to effect 50%

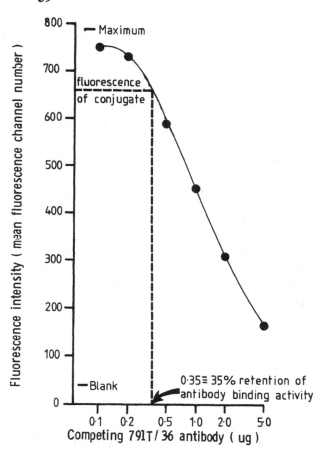

FIGURE 8. Quantitation of MTX-HSA-791T/36 binding to cells under cytotoxicity test conditions. Cells were incubated with MTX-HSA-791T/36 conjugate as in the "chronic" exposure cytotoxicity test, washed, and treated with FITC-labeled rabbit anti-HSA at 4°C. Mean fluorescence intensity was determined using a flow cytofluorimeter and plotted against methotrexate concentration of conjugate. The methotrexate concentration of conjugate at the IC_{50} of the different assays has been indicated on the binding curve.

inhibition of 791T tumor cell growth as determined by the "pre-treatment" test (15- to 30-minute incubation) requires almost saturation of the tumor cell with conjugate. However, delivery of MTX sufficient to produce IC_{50} in the "chronic exposure" or clonogenic assay occurs at about 20% saturation of tumor antigen binding sites.

3. DAUNOMYCIN-791T/36 ANTIBODY CONJUGATES

Anthracyclines represent an important class of antitumor agents with the potential for antibody targeting. Thus, conjugates of daunomycin with 791T/36 antibody were synthesized (18). Four types of daunomycin conjugates have been prepared involving either the sugar amino group or the 14-position of the drug (Fig. 9). Direct conjugation of daunomycin to 791T/36 antibody through antibody free amino groups was effected by reacting 14-bromo-daunomycin (14-bromo-Dau) to antibody (Fig. 10, conjugate 1). This conjugation procedure simply involved reacting antibody with a 25 molar excess of 14-bromo-Dau at neutral pH for 4 hours, and separation of products by chromatography on Sephadex G25. Alternatively, 14-bromo-Dau was linked to antibody through free thiol groups, thus producing a thio ether linkage. Thio groups were introduced into antibody by means of the heterobifunctional reagent N succinimidyl-3 (2-pyridyldithio) proprionate (SPDP) followed by reduction of

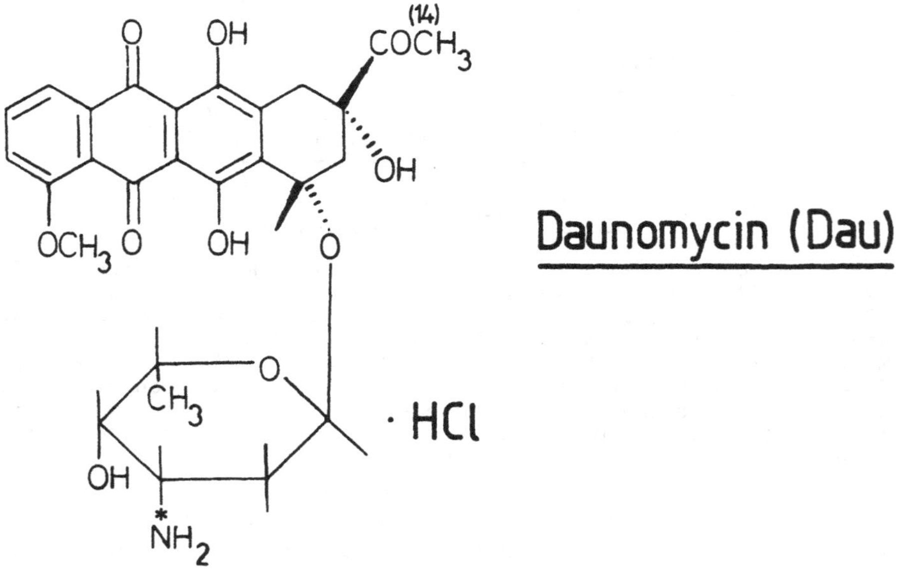

Daunomycin (Dau)

FIGURE 9. Structural formula of daunomycin hydrochloride. Conjugates with antibody were prepared with linkages either at the 14-carbon position or at the sugar amino group (*).

the dithiopyridyl (DTP) residues with dithiothreitol. The thiolated antibody was then reacted with a 10-fold molar excess of 14-bromo-Dau (with respect to DTP residues) using conditions established so that there was no reaction with free antibody.

Conjugates were also prepared by linking antibody to the sugar amino group of daunomycin (conjugates 3 and 4, Fig. 10). The sugar amino group of daunomycin was initially modified by reaction with <u>cis</u> aconitic anhydride or succinic anhydride. These derivatives were then linked to antibody using 1-ethyl-3 (3-dimethylaminopropyl) carbodiimide to effect peptide bonding using conditions which minimize antibody cross-linking. This was estimated by sodium dodecyl sulfate-polyacrylamide gel electrophoresis (SDS-PAGE) to be less than 5% (18).

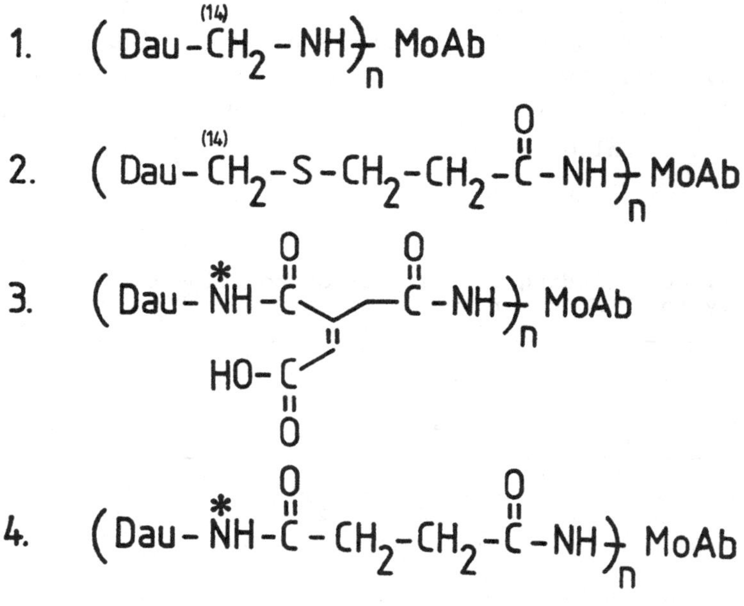

1. $\left(Dau - \overset{(14)}{C}H_2 - NH \right)_n MoAb$

2. $\left(Dau - \overset{(14)}{C}H_2 - S - CH_2 - CH_2 - \overset{O}{\overset{\|}{C}} - NH \right)_n MoAb$

3. $\left(Dau - \overset{*}{N}H - \overset{O}{\overset{\|}{C}} \diagdown \diagup \overset{O}{\overset{\|}{C}} - NH \right)_n MoAb$
   $HO - \overset{}{\underset{\overset{\|}{O}}{C}} \diagup$

4. $\left(Dau - \overset{*}{N}H - \overset{O}{\overset{\|}{C}} - CH_2 - CH_2 - \overset{O}{\overset{\|}{C}} - NH \right)_n MoAb$

FIGURE 10. Structural formula describing bond linkages between daunomycin and antibody for conjugates 1 to 4. Conjugates 1 and 2 were prepared with linkages at the 14-carbon position of the drug and conjugates 3 and 4 were prepared with linkages at the sugar amino group (*) of the drug.

Molar ratios of drug-antibody prepared by the above four procedures, as measured by spectrophotometry, ranged from 3.0 to 4.1:1. With this degree of substitution, there was high retention of 791T/36 antibody immunoreactivity in conjugates containing daunomycin linked through the 14-position. As illustrated in Table 6, conjugates 1 and 2 prepared by linking 14-bromo-Dau to free or thiolated antibody, respectively, competed as effectively as free 7891T/36 antibody with FITC-791T/36 antibody binding to tumor cells. Also, binding of both conjugates to 791T cells was comparable to that of unmodified antibody when measured by uptake under saturating conditions. In these tests cell-bound conjugates as well as unmodified antibody were detected by second antibody interactions with FITC-labeled rabbit antimouse immunoglobulin.

Conjugation of daunomycin via the sugar amino group (conjugates 3 and 4) produced a more substantial loss of 791T/36 antibody reativity. These products retained only 16-23% of 791T/36 antibody activity when tested by their capacity to compete with unlabeled antibody for 791T target cells (Table 6).

Table 6. Cell binding activity of daunomycin-791T/36 monoclonal antibody to 791T tumor cells as assessed by flow cytometry.

Conjugate number	Indirect immunofluorescence assay[a]	Competitive inhibition assay[b]
1	108 ± 25 ($n^c = 4$)	124 ± 28 ($n = 4$)
2	$68, 84$ ($n = 2$)	98 ± 17 ($n = 4$)
3	$81, 80$ ($n = 2$)	23 ± 4 ($n = 4$)
4	NT[d]	$16, 17$ ($n = 2$)

[a]Percent binding of FITC-labeled rabbit antimouse Ig antiglobulin to cell-bound conjugate compared with 791T/36 antibody.
[b]Percent recovery (mean $\pm$ SD) of the capacity of conjugate to inhibit FITC-labeled 791T/36 antibody cell-binding activity.
[c]n = number of preparations tested.
[d]NT = not tested.

The conjugate produced via the _cis_ aconityl linkage (conjugate 3) did bind to 791T tumor cells as demonstrated by reaction of conjugate-treated cells with FITC-rabbit antimouse immunoglobulin (Table 6). Moreover, this uptake was specific since the conjugate did not bind to bladder carcinoma cells which do not express the 791T/36-defined epitope (18).

In vitro cytotoxicity tests in which free daunomycin or antibody conjugates were incubated with tumor cells for 24 hours indicated that conjugate 1, in which daunomycin was directly linked to antibody, was the most reactive, showing about 10% of the level of cytotoxicity as free drug (Table 7). Conjugates 2 and 3 were also cytotoxic for tumor cells although with activities some 40-80 times less than that of the free daunomycin. This recovery of daunomycin activity following antibody coupling is comparable to that previously observed with conjugates of daunomycin linked to proteins via the methylketone side chains (19). In order to examine whether daunomycin-791T/36 antibody conjugates exhibited selectivity of action for cells bearing the 791T/36 antibody-defined antigen, 791T osteogenic sarcoma and T24 bladder carcinoma cells were incubated for 30 minutes

Table 7. Tumor cell cytotoxicity of daunomycin and daunomycin-791T/36 antibody conjugates.

Tumor cell[a]	Cytotoxicity (IC_{50} values: daunomycin µg/ml) for:				
	Daunomycin	Daunomycin-791T/36 conjugate type			
		1	2	3	4
791T osteogenic sarcoma	0.04	0.4	2.8	2.1	>10
T14 bladder carcinoma	0.05	0.5	3.2	1.5	>10
EB33 prostate carcinoma	0.04	NT	NT	1.7	<10

[a]Tumor cells incubated with drug or conjugate for 24 hours and cell survival measured by incorporation of ^{75}Se-met (18).

with each of the three types of conjugates tested. Unbound conjugate was then removed by washing, and after a 24-hour incubation cell survival was determined by the ^{75}Se-met-uptake assay (17). All three types of conjugate were cytotoxic for sarcoma 791T cells over the range of concentrations tested (Table 8). This cytotoxicity was not observed against T24 bladder carcinoma cells, which do not bind significant amounts of the conjugates.

Table 8. Specific cytotoxicity of daunomycin-791T/36 antibody conjugates.

Conjugate type	Concentration µg daunomycin/ml	Percent cytotoxicity with tumor cells	
		791T osteogenic sarcoma	T24 bladder carcinoma
1	0.1	29	0
	1	26	0
	10	100	0
	20	100	24
	40	100	100
2	0.1	0	0
	1	4	0
	10	16	0
	40	25	12
3	0.1	0	0
	1	78	0
	10	97	0
	20	98	0
	40	100	0

Tumor cells incubated with a range of doses of conjugates (expressed in terms of daunomycin content) for 30 minutes. Cells were then washed, cultured for 24 hours, and cell survival measured by incorporation of ^{75}Se-met (18).

4. VINDESINE-791T/36 ANTIBODY CONJUGATES

Vindesine (VDS) is a potent antimitotic agent and potentially is cytotoxic for all dividing cells. This property led to the synthesis of VDS conjugates with a range of monoclonal antibodies including 791T/36, anti-CEA antibodies 11.285.14 and 14.95.55, and antimelanoma antibody 96.5. The main objective was to develop conjugates able to discriminate between cells bearing or not bearing the target antigen (20). Covalent conjugates of VDS with 791T/36 and other antibodies were prepared using the general procedures for protein coupling of vinca alkaloids. Essentially, desacetylvinblastine hydrazide was converted to the azide and reacted with antibody at pH 9.0 or vindesine hemisuccinate was activated to the N-hydroxysuccinimide ester and then reacted with antibody at pH 8.6. Conjugates were purified by gel filtration on Biogel p6 and characterized by spectrometry at 270 nm and 280 nm using the appropriate extinction coefficients for each component of the conjugate. These studies indicated a substitution ratio of 6 moles VDS/mole IgG. This degree of substitution did not affect antibody binding activity, and as shown in Figure 11, VDS-791T/36 conjugate competed as effectively as unmodified antibody with FITC-791T/36, as assessed by flow cytometry.

As with the other chemotherapeutic agents, conjugation of VDS to antibody resulted in a considerable reduction of cytotoxic activity of the drug when compared with free VDS. This is illustrated in Figure 12, which shows survival of osteogenic sarcoma 791T cells following continuous exposure to VDS or VDS-791T/36 conjugate. However, linking to antibody yielded conjugates with preferential cytotoxicity for cells expressing the 791T/36 antigen. Thus, as shown in Figure 13, VDS-791T/36 conjugate was cytotoxic for 791T cells but not ovarian carcinoma PA1 cells, which do not bind the 791T/36 antibody. This is further emphasized by tests with a range of tumor cells (Table 9), where VDS-791T/36 was only cytotoxic for tumor cells which bind the antibody conjugate.

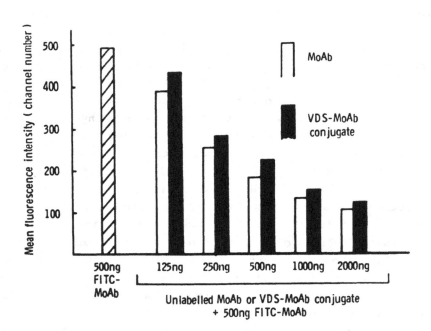

FIGURE 11. Competitive inhibition of binding of fluorescein isothiocyanate-labeled 791T/36 monoclonal antibody (FITC-MoAb) to osteosarcoma 791T cells by vindesine-conjugated antibody (VDS-MoAb) and native antibody (MoAb). FITC-MoAb binding to 791T cells measured by flow cytometry and expressed as mean fluorescence intensity (channel number)/cell.

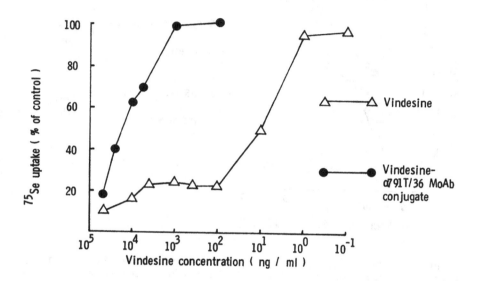

FIGURE 12. Survival of 791T osteogenic sarcoma cells cultured continuously for 24 hr with vindesine (VDS) or VDS-791T/36 monoclonal antibody conjugate (VDS-MoAb). Vertical bars indicate SE.

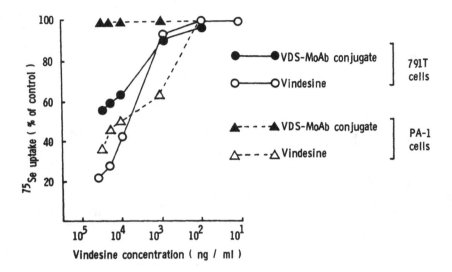

FIGURE 13. Effect of vindesine (VDS) and VDS-791T/36 monoclonal antibody on survival of tumor cells in culture. Cells were treated with the agent for 15 min, then washed and cultured for 24 hr. They were then labeled for 16 hr with ^{75}Se-met and washed 3 times. Uptake of ^{75}Se by treated cells is expressed as a percentage of that in controls (treated with phosphate-buffered saline). 791T/36, osteogenic sarcoma. PA1, ovarian carcinoma.

Table 9. Inhibition of cell survival following treatment with 791T/36-vindesine conjugate.

	Cell line	Antibody binding	Percent inhibition of ^{75}Se-met uptake at following concentration:		
			40 µg/ml	20 µg/ml	10 µg/ml
Osteogenic sarcoma	791T	++	75	73	58
	788T	++	59	36	42
	2 OS	+	77	78	90
	T 278	+	65	60	58
Melanoma	RPMI 5966	−	2	2	3
	Mel-57	−	5	10	2
Ovarian carcinoma	PA-1	−	3	4	1
Bladder carcinoma	T24	−	4	−14	0

5. THERAPEUTIC ACTIVITY OF 791T/36 MONOCLONAL ANTIBODY CONJUGATES

The therapeutic potential of 791T/36 antibody conjugates is presently evaluated against human tumor xenografts in mice immunodeprived by thymectomy, whole-body irradiation (^{60}CO-γ irradiation 9Gy), and cytosine arabinoside treatment. Although the design of these trials is far from being optimized, the initial tests indicate that antibody conjugates can suppress tumor growth. In one of the first series (20), mice implanted subcutaneously with osteogenic sarcoma 791T cells were treated twice weekly intraperitoneally with either vindesine or VDS-791T/36 conjugate (total dose of VDS 20 mg/kg). Treatment with VDS-791T/36 conjugate significantly suppressed tumor growth without any associated toxic effects (Fig. 14). Although the response to VDS was greater, the dose of compound proved toxic, with 2 of the 6 treated mice dying. This pattern of response was observed in other tests using VDS conjugated to anti-CEA monoclonal antibody (11.285.14) and antimelanoma antibody 96.5 (20). The general experience gained from these trials was that VDS-antibody conjugates retained antitumor activity. Although the antitumor activity was considerably lower than that of free

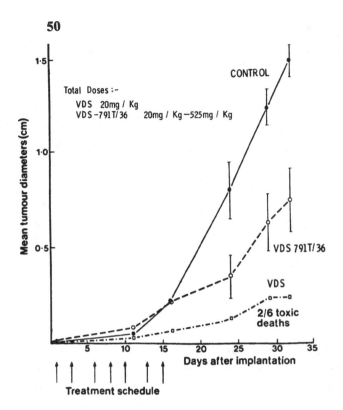

FIGURE 14. Effect of vindesine (VDS) and vindesine-791T/36 anti-body conjugate on growth of xenografts of osteogenic sarcoma 791T. Each agent was given intraperitoneally according to the treatment schedule shown. Total dose/mouse was 20 mg/kg body weight of VDS alone or conjugated to 791T/36 antibody (500 mg/kg).

VDS, this was compensated for by a marked reduction of toxicity. This is emphasized by initial acute toxicity tests with VDS and VDS-anti-CEA antibody 11.255.14. The LD_{50} for free VDS was 6.7 mg/kg, whereas no mice died following treatment with up to 90 mg/kg (as VDS) of antibody conjugate (20).

A similar experience has been gained in early trials with methotrexate conjugated to 791T/36 antibody via an HSA bridge. This is illustrated in Figure 15, which compared growth of osteo-genic sarcoma 791T in immunodeprived mice treated with MTX or MTX-HSA-791T/36 (total dose of MTX, free or conjugated, 17.5 mg/kg body weight). Using a twice weekly treatment protocol,

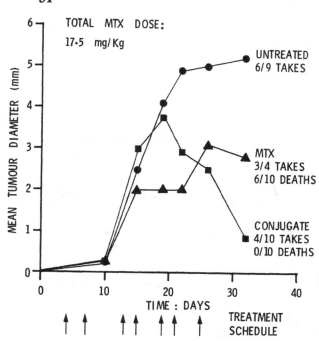

FIGURE 15. Therapy of human tumor xenografts with MTX-HSA-791T/36. Thymectomized, irradiated BALB/c mice were inoculated with $3-4 \times 10^6$ 791T cells at time 0 and treated at the indicated times with either PBS (●), 17.5 mg/kg methotrexate (▲), or 17.5 mg/kg MTX-HSA-791T/36 (■). The mean tumor diameter of those bearing tumors was plotted for each treatment and the number of animals bearing tumors over the number of animals surviving treatment is given for the relevant point.

tumors developed in 4/10 mice receiving MTX-HSA-791T/36 conjugate (control tumor growth 6/9). Considerable toxicity was observed following treatment with free MTX and 6/10 mice died. In comparison, no MTX-induced toxicity was observed in mice treated with the MTX-HSA-791T/36 conjugate.

These in vivo trials with vindesine and methotrexate linked to 791T/36 monoclonal antibody demonstrate the potential of antibody targeting of antitumor agents. But more extensive testing with respect to conjugate dose and schedule of treatment is required. It is quite clear that antibody conjugation markedly reduces drug toxicity so that the next step will be to optimize the therapeutic protocols. In this respect it is essential to

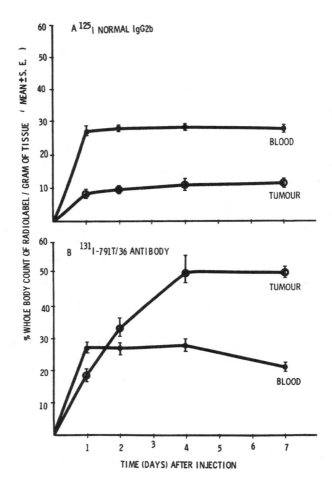

FIGURE 16. Time course of tumor and blood levels of (A) ^{125}I-normal IgG$_{2b}$ and (B) [131]I-791T/36 antibody in 791T xenograft-bearing mice. Results are expressed as % whole body counts/g tissues.

take into account the _in vivo_ pharmacokinetics of drug-antibody conjugates. This is illustrated by related investigations upon the extent and rate of deposition of radioiodine-labeled 791T/36 antibody in human tumor xenografts (16). As shown in Figure 16, following injection of ^{131}I-791T/36, localization in osteogenic sarcoma xenografts was maximum after 2 days while significant levels of radioactivity were retained for at least 5 days. Furthermore, dose-response studies indicated that tumor uptake increased over the range of 100 µg-200 µg/mouse, the maximum dose being equivalent to approximately 100 mg/kg body weight (21). As tumor became saturated with 791T/36 antibody, there was approximately 70 µg antibody/g tumor tissue. The indication from these studies is that doses of 2 mg/mouse of 791T/36 at 3- to 4-day intervals will achieve maximum tumor levels of antibody. But other factors, especially the stability of drug-antibody linkage, will have to be taken into account in designing treatment protocols. Also, drug conjugation may influence the kinetics of antibody localization, especially where drug carriers of large molecular size such as human serum albmuin are used.

6. CONCLUSIONS

There is little doubt that tumor-reactive monoclonal antibodies offer new approaches for targeting anticancer agents. There are, however, a series of interrelated developments which must be accomplished before antibody-drug targeting can be critically evaluated. This includes the selection of antibodies (or antibody fragments) with adequate tumor localizing potential, the selection of appropriate cytotoxic agents, and the design of conjugation procedures which result in both drug and antibody reactivities being maximally retained in the resulting conjugate. The investigations outlined in constructing conjugates of monoclonal antibody 791T/36 with cytotoxic drugs demonstrate that it is feasible to develop conjugates in which drug activities are retained. In most instances, however, antibody conjugation results in considerable reduction of cytotoxic activity when compared with that of the free drug. Furthermore, in general it is not feasible to introduce many drug residues into an antibody molecule without causing marked reduction in antibody reactivity. This will be dependent upon the chemical characteristics of drug moieties so that, for example, direct conjugation of more than four methotrexate residues to 791T/36 antibody could not be achieved without significantly reducing antibody reactivity, whereas at least 6 moles vindesine/mole antibody could be readily introduced without affecting antibody. From these considerations it is clear that the use of spacer molecules to which greater amounts of drug can be attached before linkage to antibody will prove advantageous. This has already been demonstrated with methotrexate-human serum albumin conjugates, but it has to be recognized that increasing the size of the drug-antibody conjugate will further impede their in vivo extravasation and tumor deposition in tumors.

The investigations described with 791T/36 antibody establish that conjugates with well-defined characteristics can be produced and this has allowed testing of their in vivo effects on human tumor xenografts. It has been shown that conjugates with vindesine and methotrexate suppress growth of osteogenic sarcoma 791T xenografts, but the true therapeutic potential of these conjugates remains to be established. In this respect the very significant reduction of drug toxicity following antibody conjugation provides a basis for dose-response studies.

Finally, the selection of monoclonal antibodies which can be used for targeting drugs will be dependent upon related investigations showing that they actually localize in human tumors. This has been established with monoclonal antibody 791T/36 in a series of investigations showing that antibody radiolabeled with ^{131}I or ^{111}In localizes in human colorectal and ovarian tumors and in osteogenic sarcomas, permitting their detection by gamma camera imaging (12-15,22). For example, in one series of 56 patients with gastrointestinal cancer, 8/11 primary colon carcinomas gave positive images with tumor to nontumor ratios of 4:1 (14). Of 15 patients with metastatic or recurrent tumors, all but 2 gave positive images following injection of ^{131}I-labeled 791T/36 antibody (14). Resected tissue samples from patients with primary colorectal cancer were also analyzed for distribution of ^{131}I radioactivity and this indicated a tumor to nontumor ratio of 2.5:1. In this series of patients (14) and also in ovarian cancer (22), 791T/36 antibody was primarily located in the stromal element of tumors and in the pseudoacini. This emphasizes the earlier comments that tumor tissue targeting rather than specific tumor cell targeting of antitumor agents can be more easily achieved. This adds a further consideration in designing drug targeting systems since biodegradable bonding of drug to antibody will ensure that agents are released in the tumor environment.

ACKNOWLEGMENTS

I would like to thank my colleagues for permission to reproduce their data.

REFERENCES

1. Baldwin RW. 1984. In: Cancer Chemotherapy Annual 6 (Eds HM Pinedo, BA Chabner), Elsevier, Amsterdam, pp 181-199.
2. Embleton MJ, Garnett MC. 1984. In: Monoclonal Antibodies for Tumour Detection and Drug Targeting (Eds RW Baldwin, VS Byers), Academic Press, London, in press.
3. Rowland GD, Simmonds RG. 1984. In: Monoclonal Antibodies for Tumour Detection and Drug Targeting (Eds RW Baldwin, VS Byers), Academic Press, London, in press.
4. Vitetta ES, Krolick KA, Miyama-Inaba WC, Cushley W, Uhri JW. 1983. Science 219:644-650.
5. Jansen FK, Laurent G, Liance MC, et al. 1984. In: Monoclonal Antibodies for Tumour Detection and Drug Targeting (Eds RW Baldwin, VS Byers), Academic Press, London, in press.
6. Tokes ZA, Rogers KE, Rembaum A. 1982. Proc Natl Acad Sci USA 79:2026.
7. Embleton MJ, Gunn B, Byers VS, Baldwin RW. 1981. Br J Cancer 43:582-587.
8. Roth JA, Restropo C, Scuderi P, Baldwin RW, Reichert CM, Hosoi S. 1984. Cancer Res 44:5320-5325.
9. Pimm MV, Embleton MJ, Perkins AC, et al. 1982. Int J Cancer 30:75-85.
10. Roe R, Robins RA, Laxton RR, Baldwin RW. 1985. Mol Immunol, in press.
11. Price MR, Campbell DG, Robins RA, Baldwin RW. 1982. Eur J Cancer Clin Oncol 19:81-90.
12. Farrands PA, Perkins AC, Pimm MV, et al. 1982. Lancet 8295:397-400.
13. Farrands PA, Perkins A, Sully L, et al. Journal of Bone and Joint Surgery 65:638-640.

14. Armitage NC, Perkins AC, Pimm MV, Farrands PA, Baldwin RW, Hardcastle JD. 1984. Br J Surgery 71:407-412.
15. Williams MR, Perkins AC, Campbell FC, et al. 1985. Clin Oncol, in press.
16. Garnett MC, Embleton MJ, Jacobs E, Baldwin RW. 1983. Int J Cancer 31:661-670.
17. Embleton MJ, Rowland GRF, Simmonds RG, Jacobs E, Marsden CH, Baldwin RW. 1983. Br J Cancer 47:43-39.
18. Gallego J, Price MR, Baldwin RW. 1984. Int J Cancer 33:737-744.
19. Zunino F, Gambetta R, Vigevani A, Penco S, Geroni C, DiMarco A. 1981. Tumori 67:521-524.
20. Rowland GF, Axton CA, Baldwin RW, et al. 1985. Cancer Immunol Immunother, in press.
21. Pimm MV, Baldwin RW. 1984. Eur J Cancer Clin Oncol 20:515-524.
22. Symonds EM, Perkins AC, Pimm MV, Baldwin RW, Hardy JD, Williams DA. 1984. Br J Obstet Gynaecol, in press.

3. MONOCLONAL ANTIBODIES DIRECTED TOWARDS GROWTH-RELATED RECEPTORS ON HUMAN TUMORS*

CAROL L. MACLEOD, HIDEO MASUI, IAN S. TROWBRIDGE and JOHN MENDELSOHN

1. INTRODUCTION

The potential therapeutic uses of monoclonal antibodies in the treatment of cancer have attracted considerable interest. Attention has been focused upon two approaches: 1) Serotherapy, which relies upon the host immunological effector mechanisms to eliminate antibody-coated tumor cells, and 2) antibody-toxin conjugates which selectively target covalently bound drugs or toxins to malignant tissue. We have explored a third general approach to cancer therapy, which utilizes monoclonal antibodies that act as pharmacological agents to directly block biological functions essential for cell proliferation. Cell proliferation and differentiation can be regulated by extracellular signals such as hormones and growth factors. The biochemical mechanisms by which hormonal agents influence such complex biological responses are being actively investigated in a number of laboratories.

The potential clinical utility of antireceptor antibodies is supported by both clinical and experimental evidence. Rare autoimmune diseases have been described in which antibodies either block receptor binding to its ligand or stimulate the receptor by mimicking the natural ligand: e.g., the insulin receptor in insulin-resistant diabetes (1,2), the nicotinic acetylcholine receptor in myasthenia gravis (3,4), the thyroid-stimulating hormone receptor in Graves' disease (5) and in primary myxedema (6).

*This work was supported by NIH grants CA33397, CA23052, CA34077, CA34787, and CA17733 and by the CRCC. C.L.M. and H.M. received support from the Clayton Foundation.

K.A. Foon and A.C. Morgan, Jr. (eds.), *Monoclonal Antibody Therapy of Human Cancer.* Copyright © 1985. Martinus Nijhoff Publishing, Boston. All rights reserved.

A number of antireceptor antibodies have been obtained in order to study hormone receptor interactions and to examine their effects on cellular proliferation in vitro and in vivo. Antibodies to β-adrenergic receptors have been experimentally developed by a number of investigators (7-9). Antibodies to the receptor for prolactin have been obtained from guinea pigs (10) and monoclonal antibodies to the complex acetylcholine receptor have also been characterized (11).

Polyclonal antibodies to human epidermal growth factor (EGF) receptors, which block binding of ^{125}I-EGF to receptor and prevent stimulation of DNA synthesis by EGF, have been described (12). Other investigators have described monoclonal antibodies against the EGF receptor which have agonist and antagonist effects upon cell functions (13).

We have demonstrated antiproliferative effects in vitro (14, 16,17) and in vivo (15,18) of anti-EGF-receptor monoclonal antibodies and antitransferrin receptor monoclonal antibodies. These experiments provide the first evidence that monoclonal antibodies directed against growth-related cell surface receptors may directly inhibit tumor cell growth by depriving tumor cells of nutritionally critical molecules or growth stimulatory signals.

Proliferating cells require a number of factors and hormones in order to be cultured in serum-free medium (19-21). Comparative studies in supplemented serum-free medium indicate that different cell types require different combinations of added factors and hormones. Cells deprived of one of these essential growth-promoting factors proliferate more slowly or in some cases become quiescent. Most receptors for essential growth factors are surface membrane receptors and potentially are antigenic targets accessible to monoclonal antibodies. Although such receptors are not known to differ from one cell type to another, the constellation of receptors present on a given cell type may be relatively unique, and thus combinations of monoclonal antibodies against specific receptors may be highly selective for some tumors.

In this chapter we review studies using antibodies developed in our laboratories against the human EGF receptor and the human and murine transferrin receptors. We briefly describe the properties of the receptors against which these antibodies are directed and summarize our findings on the inhibition of tumor growth in xenografts and transplantable murine tumors in the in vivo model systems.

2. THE EGF RECEPTOR

Specific saturable receptors for EGF are present on a wide variety of tissues including corneal cells, human fibroblasts, lens glial cells, epidermoid carcinomas, granulosa cells, vascular endothelial cells, and choriocarcinomas (22,23).

EGF is a potent mitogen for certain cultured cells and has been used extensively as a model for studying growth control (24,25). In the intact animal and in organ culture EGF appears only to stimulate the growth of epidermal and epithelial cells. However, in tissue culture EGF is mitogenic for a wide variety of cells as noted above. The cell surface EGF receptors must be occupied over an extended period to exert their mitogenic effect. If EGF is removed 4 hours after addition, no increase in cellular DNA synthesis occurs (24,26) and maximal stimulation occurs approximately 24 hours after addition of EGF. Following EGF-receptor binding the occupied receptors cluster in clathrin-coated pits, are internalized into endocytotic vesicles, and ultimately are degraded in lysosomes (27). Although the initial hormone-receptor interactions at the plasma membrane are required to obtain a biological response, the relevance of internalization of the hormone-receptor complex into the cell and the fate of the internalized receptor remain unclear (23,27).

The complete amino acid sequence of the EGF receptor has been obtained by sequencing cDNA from the human epidermoid carcinoma cell line A431 (28,29) which overexpresses the receptor (2-3 x 10^6 molecules/cell) (30). The receptor is a 170-kilodalton glycoprotein comprised of a single polypeptide chain which spans the cytoplasmic membrane. The aminoterminal 621 residues on the external face of the plasma membrane contain the EGF binding region and are glycosylated at several sites. A hydrophobic portion between residues 621 and 644 is the likely transmembrane region (28,31). The C-terminal 542 residues comprise the internal cytoplasmic portion of the EGF receptor containing the tyrosine kinase activity, which is stimulated by EGF binding (28,31). Since the EGF receptor kinase phosphorylates tyrosine residues, this normal growth-regulating system bears a similarity to the mechanism employed by some oncogenic viruses to transform normal cellular growth controls (32).

The EGF receptor kinase autophosphorylates the EGF receptor at three sites near the carboxyterminus (33) and phosphorylates itself and other cellular substrates at tyrosine residues (34, 36-39), which is a property shared by the insulin receptor (40,41). Furthermore, the receptor serves as a substrate for protein kinase C (the TPA receptor) (35) which phosphorylates the EGF receptor at threonine residues. Interestingly, when the EGF receptor functions as a substrate and is phosphorylated by protein kinase C, the receptor kinase activity of the receptor is inhibited (35). Recently, the kinase domain of the EGF receptor was found to be highly homologous to the v-erb-b oncogene (28,36). The recent discovery that transforming growth factor alpha binds to the EGF receptor and induces phosphorylation of tyrosine in the EGF receptor further underscores the importance of growth factor receptors in malignant cell proliferation. One possible mechanism of malignant transformation that has been suggested is that tumor cells may have the ability to stimulate their own proliferation through the "autocrine" secretion of a transforming growth factor. Such factors bind to cell receptors for normal growth factors expressed on the tumor cell surface (42-44). The identification of the EGF receptor as an expressed c-erb-b proto-oncogene provides an indication that regulation of responses to growth factors may provide a novel method for inhibiting tumor cell proliferation.

2.1. Production of monoclonal antibodies to the human EGF
receptor

A431 human epidermoid carcinoma cells lend themselves to the
study of EGF-receptor interactions and are a good source of
antigens for the production of antibodies because they have an
extremely high number of EGF receptors ($1-3 \times 10^6$/cell) (30).
BALB/c mice were immunized with A431 EGF receptors which had
been partially purified on EGF-affigel as described (45). Splenocytes were fused with NS-1-Ag4-1 murine myeloma cells according
to the method of Galfre et al. (46). The first assay used to
identify anti-EGF-receptor monoclonal antibodies was to test
whether the hybridoma culture supernatants contained antibodies
that bound to the surface of A431 cells using ^{125}I-rabbit antimouse IgG in an antibody-binding assay. Supernatants which
were positive were then tested for their capacity to inhibit
binding of ^{125}I-EGF to A431 cells. At this stage, hybridomas
were cloned and then immunoprecipitation studies with purified
monoclonal antibodies were carried out to determine which
antibodies could immunoprecipitate EGF receptors from solubil-
ized A431 membranes. This procedure showed that monoclonal
antibody 455, which bound to A431 cells but did not block
binding of ^{125}I-EGF, nevertheless reacted with a surface protein
which has the capacity to autophosphorylate and comigrates with
authentic EGF receptor.

2.2. Properties of monoclonal antibodies against the EGF
receptor

From the initial series of fusions, four anti-EGF-receptor
monoclonal antibodies were obtained. The antibodies were characterized by measuring their binding to A431 cells and their ability
to inhibit binding of each other and of EGF (Table 1) (47). Each
of the four antibodies and EGF itself gave similar estimates for
the number of EGF receptors on A431 cells (approximately $2-3 \times$
10^6 binding sites/cell). The apparent K_D's of monoclonal antibodies 528, 225, and 579 were comparable to that of EGF, in the
range of 1-3 nM, whereas the affinity of antibody 455 was about
20 nM. The three high-affinity antibodies and EGF were able to

Table 1. Monoclonal antibody characteristics.

| | A431 binding | | % inhibition of binding by 100 nM ligand | |
Ligand	K_D (x 10^9 M)	Sites/cell (x 10^{-6})	^{125}I-EGF	^{125}I-528
528 IgG$_{2a}$	2.0	1.6	100	100
225 IgG$_1$	0.9	1.5	100	100
579 IgG$_{2a}$	1.5	1.2	100	100
455 IgG$_1$	20	1.8	0	0
EGF	2-5	1.5-3.0	100	95

Details of the procedures used to obtain these data are found in reference 47.

block binding of ^{125}I-EGF completely, whereas 455 IgG failed to block EGF binding. EGF blocked nearly all binding of ^{125}I-528 antibody. None of the antibodies reacted with EGF (47).

The inhibition of EGF binding by antireceptor monoclonal antibodies was characterized by measuring binding of EGF at various concentrations in the presence of a constant concentration of antibody. Double reciprocal plots of the data showed that inhibition of EGF binding by 528 IgG was primarily competitive (48). Similar results were obtained with 225 IgG and 579 IgG (48).

Almost 30 anti-EGF-receptor monoclonal antibodies obtained by Schlessinger's, Waterfield's, and our groups have been examined for their carbohydrate specificity (49,50). All except three blocking antibodies, 255, 528, and 579, recognize carbohydrate structures. 455 is the only one developed in our laboratory which recognized an oligosaccharide, a blood group A-related structure. Because the EGF-blocking antibodies inhibited proliferation of some cells (see below) and bound to human EGF-bearing cells of several sources, they provided powerful and unique reagents to study the receptor and to attempt to specifically modulate receptor functions.

The monoclonal anti-EGF antibodies 225, 528, and 579 reacted efficiently with other human cells bearing EGF receptors, including human foreskin fibroblasts and a variety of tumor cell lines. This was in contrast to the majority of monoclonal antibodies obtained against the A431 EGF receptor which did not recognize the receptor on other human cell types. However, the antibodies were species-specific and did not react with murine or rat cell lines bearing EGF receptors (47). Since EGF itself is not species-specific, the three EGF antibodies that block EGF binding are probably reacting with antigenic determinants close to, but not directly at, the binding site for EGF.

2.3. Antiproliferative effects of anti-EGF-receptor monoclonal antibodies upon cultured cells

The biological effect of anti-EGF-receptor monoclonal antibodies on cell proliferation was investigated using cell lines grown in supplemented serum-free culture medium. Human foreskin fibroblasts required EGF for optimum proliferation in the absence of serum. Anti-EGF receptor antibodies 528, 225, and 579 inhibited EGF-stimulated human foreskin fibroblast proliferation in a dose-dependent manner, whereas 455 had no effect (14,47). The slow rate of proliferation observed in serum-free culture, in the absence of added EGF, was not further inhibited by any of the anti-EGF monoclonal antibodies. Similarly, a variety of tumor cell lines were stimulated to proliferate in serum-free culture by the addition of EGF (Table 2). EGF-induced stimulation was inhibited by monoclonal antibodies 528, 225, or 579 (15,47). In contrast to most cells bearing EGF receptors, the growth of A431 cells was inhibited by the addition of nM amounts of EGF (51,52). Although the detailed mechanism(s) of inhibition is not known, it may be related to the extraordinary number of EGF receptors on these cells. When the anti-EGF-receptor monoclonal antibodies were incubated with A431 cells in serum-free defined medium without EGF, each of the three blocking antibodies (528, 225, and 579) inhibited cell growth in a dose-dependent manner (47). Higher relative concentrations of 528 IgG Fab fragments also partially inhibited cellular proliferation.

Table 2. Studies of human tumor cells in culture and in xenografts.

Cells*	In vivo effects upon proliferation†		Relative receptor number on cultured cells	Effect of treating xenografts with 528 IgG‡
	EGF	528 IgG		
NFF	S§	N	Low‖	–
A431	I	I	High	I
T222	I	I	Low	I
T423	I	I	Low	I
HeLa	S	N	Low	N
Li-7	N	N	Low	N
Li-7A	I	I	High	I
T323	S	N	Low	N
T84	N	N	Low	N
T24	S	N	Low	N
T293	S	N	Low	N

*The cell types are as follows: NFF = normal foreskin fibroblasts; A431 = vulvar epidermoid carcinoma; T222 = lung epidermoid carcinoma; T423 = epidermoid carcinoma (ear); HeLa = cervical adenocarcinoma; Li-7 = hepatoma; Li-7A = hepatoma (variant); T323 = epidermoid carcinoma (larynx); T84 = colon carcinoma; T24 = astrocytoma; T293 = oat cell carcinoma.
†Cells were cultured in serum-free medium or 0.5% serum-supplemented medium. Proliferation was assayed in the presence or absence of 30 nM EGF or 10 and 100 nM 528 IgG by comparing the cell counts after 5 days of culture in the presence or absence of IgG.
‡Mice bearing xenografts were treated intraperitoneally twice weekly with 2 mg 528 IgG, for 3-6 weeks, as described (15).
§I = inhibits; N = no effect; S = stimulates
‖Low = low (typical) number (3-5 x 10^4); High = high number (0.5-2 x 10^6).

Both EGF and antibody 528 inhibited cell proliferation of three additional tumor cell lines, two epidermal in origin and one derived from a hepatoma (Table 2). The Li-7A line was cloned, without any deliberate selective pressures, from Li-7 hepatoma cells which are neither inhibited by EGF nor by anti-EGF-receptor antibody. The data showing differential effects of EGF upon Li-7 and Li-7A hepatoma cells are presented in Figure 1. Similar inhibition occurred when Li-7A cells were exposed to 528 IgG or 225 IgG in culture. The fact that Li-7A

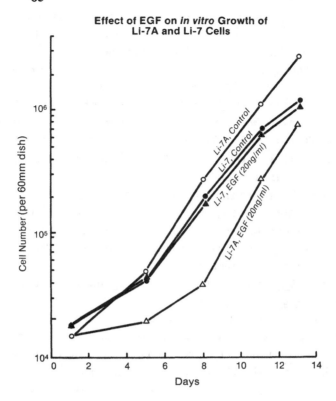

Effect of EGF on *in vitro* Growth of Li-7A and Li-7 Cells

FIGURE 1. Effects of EGF upon cultured hepatoma cells. Two x 10^4 Li-7 or Li-7A cells were plated in DME:F12 (1:1) medium supplemented with 0.5% newborn calf serum. On the following day, the medium was replaced with fresh medium, and the EGF was added to the appropriate cultures at a concentration of 20 ng/ml. Medium was changed on Day 4, and the cell number was counted in a Coulter Counter.

cells clearly differed from Li-7 cells in their responsiveness to EGF and in their receptor number (Table 2) suggested the potential importance of tumor cell heterogeneity in planning for therapy with antireceptor antibodies.

In cell lines inhibited by EGF, the blocking monoclonal antibodies appeared to mimic the action of EGF in suppressing cell proliferation. However, the antibodies failed to elicit increased phosphorylation of the EGF receptor in A431 cells (see below) and therefore could not be considered agonistic effectors. In addition, the blocking antibodies were not intrinsically inhibitory to the proliferation of cells stimulated by EGF. Rather, they reversed the stimulatory effect of EGF.

The data in Table 2 show that the inhibition of cellular proliferation by EGF or by EGF-blocking antireceptor antibodies occurred in cells with increased numbers of EGF receptors and also in T222 and T423 cells which have normal receptor numbers, in the range of 3×10^4/cell. The mechanism by which anti-EGF-receptor antibodies blocked proliferation of the same group of cells which are also inhibited by EGF is unclear at this time. It would be interesting to determine whether differences in receptor turnover kinetics, phosphorylation activity, or structure may account for the unusual property of EGF-induced and antibody-induced inhibition.

2.4. Antiproliferative effects of monoclonal antibodies upon tumor xenografts

In order to determine an effective schedule of monoclonal antibody treatment to be used in our in vivo experiments, the clearance of anti-EGF-receptor monoclonal antibodies was examined. ^{125}I-labeled 528 IgG was injected intraperitoneally into athymic mice carrying A431 tumors, and the serum level of radioactivity was measured daily. One mg of ^{125}I-528 IgG had a half-life of 3 days in vivo (15), suggesting that a twice per week treatment schedule would be satisfactory.

Intraperitoneal injection of 2 mg of anti-EGF-receptor antibody completely inhibited A431 tumor formation when tumor cells were injected the same day the antibody treatment was started (15). Furthermore, no tumor was detectable in these mice for 2 months following the end of treatment. Pathologic examination of necropsy specimens after 2 months revealed no evidence of residual tumor cells. Treatment with equimolar amounts of EGF did not produce inhibition of tumor growth. Control unrelated monoclonal antibody or mouse serum immunoglobulin had no effect on tumor growth.

Surprisingly, 455 IgG, which lacks EGF-blocking activity and had no effect on A431 cell proliferation in tissue culture, resulted in inhibition of A431 tumor growth (47). Complete inhibition of A431 tumor formation by 225 IgG and 455 IgG required 2 mg per injection, whereas 0.2 mg of 528 IgG per treatment was effective in inhibiting A431 xenograft growth (15).

The ability of monoclonal antibody treatment to inhibit the growth of established tumors was also assessed. When A431 tumors had grown to an approximate volume of 1 cm^3, twice weekly injections of 528 IgG were initiated. The same schedule and dose which were effective against freshly inoculated tumor cells reduced the tumor growth rate significantly but tumors failed to regress (15).

The ability of 528 IgG to inhibit the proliferation of the human tumors listed in Table 2 was examined. Xenografts of HeLa cells, T323 cells, and Li-7 hepatoma tumor cells, which were not inhibited from proliferating in serum-free culture by EGF or by anti-EGF-receptor monoclonal antibodies, were similarly resistant to any inhibitory effect of antibody in vivo. In contrast, the four tumors which were inhibited by monoclonal antibody in culture were also inhibited when implanted as xenografts and treated with anti-EGF-receptor antibodies (Table 2). As noted in Figure 1, the Li-7A cell line was more inhibited by EGF than the parent Li-7 hepatoma cell line from which it was cloned. The data showing differential effects of anti-EGF receptor antibody on Li-7 and Li-7A hepatoma cell xenografts are presented in Figure 2 and illustrate that a malignancy other than an epidermoid carcinoma can be effectively treated with anti-EGF-receptor monoclonal antibodies. Several other cell lines established from two lung adenocarcinomas and an embryonal carcinoma, an ovarian carcinoma, and a colon carcinoma were unresponsive to treatment with 528 IgG when grown as xenografts in nude mice. These unresponsive tumors have not yet been tested in vitro because they are not yet fully adapted to growth in culture. Each of the tumors which was inhibited as a xenograft was also inhibited by EGF and antireceptor antibody in culture. Future experiments will attempt to determine the explanation for this observation.

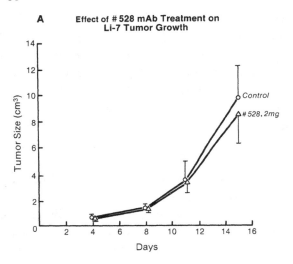

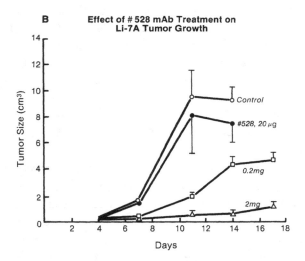

FIGURE 2. Effects of anti-EGF-receptor monoclonal antibody upon xenografts of hepatoma cell lines: (A) Li-7 hepatoma; (B) Li-7A, a cloned variant. Treatment with various doses of 528 IgG intraperitoneally, twice weekly, was begun on the day of tumor cell inoculation. Tumor size was measured in 6 animals for each experimental variable (mean + SEM). The dose-dependent inhibition of Li-7A growth is contrasted with the lack of effect on Li-7 at the highest antibody concentration (2 mg/treatment).

The data from in vivo studies of xenografts shown in Table 2 raise interesting questions about the mechanism of the antitumor activity for anti-EGF-receptor monoclonal antibodies. Most but not all inhibited tumors are epidermoid in origin. The presence of EGF receptors on cells was not sufficient for inhibition, since a large number of EGF receptor-bearing human tumor cell lines were not prevented from growing as xenografts (Table 2). The presence of high receptor numbers appeared to be unnecessary, since cultured T222 and T423 cells had normal receptor content. However, neither the in vivo receptor number nor the number of in vivo immunoreactive sites had been determined. Since a recent report presented evidence that a variety of human tumor cells show a high number of EGF receptors in situ (53,54), it is possible that T222 and T423 cells may display increased EGF receptors in vivo. We postulate that this could occur if, when cells from some xenografts are established in culture, there were a selection for reduced receptor number. Alternatively, the intense keratinization observed around some cultured epidermoid cells may interfere with the measurement of EGF receptors and lead to an underestimate of receptor number. Alternatively, T222 and T423 tumor cells may express a low number of EGF receptors in vivo (comparable to in vitro), and the mechanism of 528 IgG-induced inhibition of tumor cells in vivo may be unrelated to receptor number. To explore this question further, we have recently developed a radioimmunoassay for measuring receptor numbers in tumor xenografts.

It should be mentioned that Koprowski et al. have produced some monoclonal antibodies against human tumor-associated antigens which inhibit the growth of these tumors in athymic mice (55). All monoclonal antibodies with antitumor activity were of the IgG_{2a} isotype. The results were interpreted to indicate that the antitumor activity was accomplished via macrophage-mediated cytotoxicity. However, 255 IgG is of the IgG_1 isotype (47), indicating the possibility that more than one mechanism may be responsible for tumor cell inhibition in vivo.

The fact that 455 IgG inhibited proliferation of grafted A431 cells, but had much less effect on A431 cells in tissue culture, raised additional questions about the mechanism of tumor inhibition in vivo. Further experiments must be performed to test: 1) whether 455 IgG blocks proliferation of tumor cell xenografts which display a normal number of EGF receptors; 2) whether the ineffectiveness of 455 IgG to inhibit cellular proliferation in culture is due to a weaker affinity for the EGF receptor, compared with the three blocking antibodies; 3) whether the 455 IgG is internalized poorly or alters the kinetics of receptor internalization or processing; 4) whether 455 IgG inhibition of tumor cell growth in xenografts is due to a nonspecific cellular cytotoxicity elicited by the presence of bound IgG with exposed Fc fragments (but, if so, why is in vivo inhibition limited to only a subset of tumors bearing EGF receptors?).

2.5. Anti-EGF-receptor monoclonal antibodies' effect on EGF-stimulated autophosphorylation

Changes in cellular phosphorylation, particularly upon tyrosine residues, have been associated with several cellular transforming oncogenes and with alterations in cellular growth control. Anti-EGF-receptor monoclonal antibodies are useful reagents to examine EGF receptor-induced tyrosine kinase. The antibodies were used to alter the concentration of EGF receptors available for kinase stimulation by EGF in order to quantitate EGF-induced autophosphorylation by immunoprecipitating EGF receptors (45). Further, they were used in experiments to show that autophosphorylation is an intramolecular reaction (57).

The effects of EGF and antireceptor monoclonal antibody 528 upon the phosphorylation of the EGF receptor and other cellular substrates revealed that EGF increased the phosphotyrosine content of A431 cell total protein about 4-fold. Addition of 528 IgG inhibited the EGF-stimulated increase and did not, by itself, stimulate EGF receptor autophosphorylation in intact cells (48). 455 IgG did not affect EGF receptor protein phosphorylation either when added alone or with EGF.

2.6. Effect of anti-EGF-receptor antibodies on receptor down-regulation and internalization

An anti-EGF-receptor antibody which blocks EGF binding (225) was examined for its effect upon the surface expression of EGF receptors. The antibody was compared with EGF for its ability to induce down-regulation. EGF and 225 reduced the available EGF surface receptors (down-regulation) to a similar extent (56). Since 225 appeared to induce down-regulation of the EGF receptor, we compared the rate of ^{125}I-labeled 225 and 455 in intact A431 cells. The results suggested that 225 was internalized and degraded to a similar extent and with similar kinetics as was EGF. In contrast, 455 IgG appeared to be degraded much more slowly (56).

3. TRANSFERRIN RECEPTORS

Iron plays an important role in cell growth and metabolism. Many key reactions in energy metabolism and DNA synthesis are catalyzed by iron-containing enzymes. Under physiological conditions, however, iron in insoluble. To combat this problem, all organisms have developed transport systems to maintain iron in a soluble form and sequester it into the cell. The cellular iron transport system used by vertebrates involves the specific interaction of the iron-binding serum protein, transferrin, with a specific cell surface receptor which then facilitates iron transport across the cell membrane.

Until a few years ago, work on transferrin receptors was focused upon the maturing cells of the erythroid lineage which have a high iron requirement for heme synthesis and the placental trophoblast which channels iron to the developing embryo from the maternal circulation (58-60). Within the last 5 years, evidence was obtained indicating that many other cell types also express transferrin receptors and concomitantly it was recognized that proliferating cells expressed much larger numbers of receptors than resting cells. A wide variety of cultured human tumor cell lines express large amounts of transferrin receptors (61,62), and although transferrin receptors were not detectable on normal resting peripheral blood lymphocytes, after mitogenic stimulation with phytohemagglutinin, large numbers of transferrin receptors were found on the proliferating blast cells (63). This was the existing state of knowledge about the transferrin receptor at the time monoclonal antibodies against the receptor were identified (64,65). The recognition of the relationship between the expression of transferrin receptors and cell growth together with the development of monoclonal antibodies against the human transferrin receptor has permitted the application of novel methods to regulating cell growth.

3.1. Antitransferrin receptor monoclonal antibodies

Monoclonal antibodies against the transferrin receptor were obtained by several groups characterizing the cell surface differentiation antigens of human hematopoietic cells (64-66). A monoclonal antibody designated B3/25, obtained in our laboratory, reacted with a major human cell surface glycoprotein selectively expressed on actively growing cells. This molecule was subsequently shown to be the transferrin receptor in experiments that demonstrated that transferrin could be specifically coprecipitated as a complex with the cell surface glycoprotein recognized by B3/25 monoclonal antibody (67). Similar observations were also made with the monoclonal antibody OKT9 (68,69). With the aid of monoclonal antibodies, the transferrin receptor of human cells has been extensively characterized. The receptor, the bulk of which is exposed on the cell surface, is a transmembrane glycoprotein (Mr = 200,000) consisting of two identical disulfide-bonded subunits (70,71). The structure of transferrin receptors of other species is similar to that of the human transferrin receptor (72).

Recently, considerable progress has been made in understanding how transferrin receptors mediate iron uptake into the cell (73,74). The major features of this process are that transferrin receptors, bound to transferrin, are endocytosed via coated pits (75-77) and within a few minutes are found in endosomes. Acidification of endosomes causes dissociation of iron from transferrin, and transferrin receptors still complexed with apotransferrin are recycled back to the cell surface. Under neutral conditions found at the cell surface, apotransferrin rapidly dissociates from the transferrin receptor allowing the receptor to participate in another round of iron uptake. The half-life of the receptor-ligand complex on the cell surface is about 5 minutes, and the entire recycling process takes about 20 minutes (75). The half-life of transferrin receptors on human cells is approximately 1-3 days. Clearly, very little degradation of the transferrin receptor occurs during each round of recycling.

3.2. Expression of transferrin receptors on normal tissues and tumor cells in vivo

The original observations linking the expression of trans-ferrin receptors to cell proliferation were made by studying the cell growth in vitro (61,62,67,69). However, it is now well documented that this relationship is also found in vivo. Further, some tumors express substantially larger numbers of transferrin receptors relative to normal tissues. Early studies (78,79) suggested that transferrin receptors are expressed on breast carcinomas to a much greater extent than on normal breast tissue. These initial observations have now been extended by more recent studies using monoclonal antibodies directed against the human transferrin receptor. The distribution of transferrin receptors was examined in a wide range of normal and malignant human tissues using four different monoclonal antibodies to the transferrin receptor of human cells (80). In normal tissues, transferrin receptors were found only in a limited number of sites, notably basal epidermis, testis, liver, and pancreas. In contrast to this limited expression in normal tissue, the receptor was widely distributed in carcinomas, sarcomas, and in lymphoid biopsies from Hodgkin's disease patients. Of a total of 87 samples of malignant tissue tested for transferrin receptors by immunoperoxidase staining of cryostat sections, 70 were found to be positive. Further, a variable proportion of the malignant cells from cases of acute leukemia expressed transferrin receptors (64,65,67,68). In particular, a large fraction of cells from a majority of T-cell leukemias express large numbers of transferrin receptors. Studies of the trans-ferrin receptor expression on B-cell lymphomas (81-83) have

shown that high expression of transferrin receptors is correlated with high-grade lymphomas and with increased rates of
cell proliferation. A correlation between the expression of
transferrin receptors and patient survival suggests that the
expression of transferrin receptors may be of prognostic value
in that group of diseases.

The transferrin receptors in the mouse and rat show essentially similar distribution as has been found in man. The
distribution of transferrin receptors on pluripotent hematopoietic stem cells has been examined in animal studies. If
transferrin receptors were expressed on such cells, then hematopoietic tissue damage would be expected to limit the use of
antitransferrin receptor antibodies in immunotherapy. However,
ablation experiments in the mouse employing antitransferrin
receptor antibody-ricin A conjugates (84) and cell sorting
experiments in the rat gave concordant results and showed
that the pluripotential hematopoietic stem cell derived from
bone marrow and fetal liver is transferrin receptor negative
(W. Jeffries and A.F. Williams, unpublished results).

3.3. Monoclonal antibodies that block transferrin receptor
function

The monoclonal antibodies originally obtained against the
transferrin receptor of human cells did not interfere significantly with receptor function. We sought to identify such an
antibody by purifying the transferrin receptor from detergent
extracts of the human T-cell leukemic cell lines CCRF-CEM by
affinity chromatography utilizing a B3/25 monoclonal antibody-
Sepharose column. Mice were then immunized with the purified
glycoprotein, and from the fusions of spleen cells from these
immunized mice hybridomas were assayed for the production of
monoclonal antibodies that blocked the binding of transferrin
to the leukemic cell line. This approach led to the identification of one monoclonal antibody designated 42/6 which had the
desired properties (85). This antibody has been shown to inhibit the transferrin-mediated uptake of iron by CCRF-CEM cells
by more than 90%. The purified monoclonal antibody also inhibited the growth of CCRF-CEM leukemic cells and PHA-stimulated

human peripheral blood lymphocytes in vitro (17,85). Prolonged exposure of the cells to monoclonal antibody 42/6 caused the arrest of the cells in S phase of the cell cycle. These results provided the first evidence that monoclonal antibodies can be used directly as pharmacological agents to directly regulate the growth of tumor cells.

We were interested in the question of whether monoclonal antibodies that block transferrin receptor function could be used as therapeutic agents in vivo in the treatment of malignant disease. However, since transferrin receptors are expressed on proliferating cells in normal tissues, the toxicity of in vivo administered transferrin receptor monoclonal antibody should be assessed in an animal model system. For this reason, we sought a monoclonal antibody against the murine transferrin receptor with properties similar to that of 42/6 monoclonal antibody. From a library of over 8,000 rat monoclonal antibodies against mouse hematopoietic cells and tumor cell lines, a monoclonal antibody designated RI7 208 was identified which reacted with the murine transferrin receptor and inhibited its function (86). It was shown that this antibody could inhibit the growth of murine hematopoietic cell lines in vitro and was therefore a candidate for use in model immunotherapy experiments.

3.4. Immunotherapy with antimouse transferrin receptor antibody RI7 208 in vivo

For initial immunotherapy experiments, the transplantable AKR mouse T-cell leukemia SL-2 was chosen as a model system. Several factors were taken into consideration when making this choice. First, this leukemic cell line had been used to investigate the requirements for effective serotherapy with anti-Thy-1.1 monoclonal antibodies (87,88). Such studies provided a standard against which to compare the antitumor activity of antitransferrin receptor antibodies in vivo. Second, this model was also attractive in that if therapeutic effects were obtained with the transplantable T-cell leukemia, studies could then be extended to include spontaneous T-cell leukemia in AKR mice. Third, it is known that T-cell leukemias in man frequently express high numbers of transferrin receptors and that the in vitro growth of human T-leukemic cell lines is particularly sensitive to the effects of the murine monoclonal antibody 42/6, which blocks transferrin-mediated iron uptake. Consequently, T-cell leukemia might be expected to be an appropriate starting point for attempting immunotherapy with antitransferrin receptor antibodies in clinical studies. Finally, a long-term objective is to use antireceptor antibodies such as the antitransferrin receptor antibodies that block function in combination with other monoclonal antibodies 1) against the EGF receptor as discussed above, or 2) against differentiation antigens and tumor-associated antigens that mediate antitumor effects by activating immunological effector mechanisms. As Bernstein and his colleagues had identified the anti-Thy-1.1 monoclonal antibody designated 19E12 (88) that produced significant therapeutic effects in mice bearing the SL-2 leukemia, this model could be used to investigate the effectiveness of immunotherapy with combinations of monoclonal antibodies which induce antitumor effects by different mechanisms.

In vitro growth of SL-2 mouse leukemia cells is profoundly inhibited by the antimurine transferrin receptor antibody, RI7 208. The addition of 5 µg/ml of monoclonal antibody to cultures of SL-2 cells almost completely inhibited cell growth. The standard protocol for in vivo immunotherapy has been to inoculate groups of 6-10 mice with 1×10^6 SL-2 cells subcutaneously and then inject various amounts of purified monoclonal antibodies either intravenously or intraperitoneally. Both the rate of growth of the primary tumors in control and antibody-treated mice and their survival was followed. The results of two trials, shown in Figure 3, illustrate the major observations that have been made to date. The monoclonal antitransferrin receptor antibody RI7 208, which inhibits receptor function, not only prolonged the survival time of tumor-bearing mice (Fig. 3) but also inhibited tumor growth at the primary site (Fig. 4). In contrast, another monoclonal antibody against the murine transferrin receptor which did not block receptor function did not significantly increase the survival time of tumor-bearing mice and had much less effect on growth of the primary tumor.

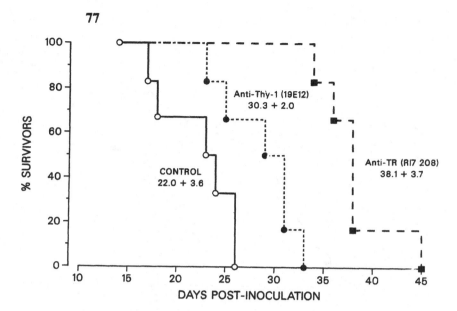

FIGURE 3. Treatment of AKR mice with rat antimurine transferrin receptor antibody, RI7 208, prolongs survival of mice challenged with SL-2 leukemia cells. A group of 6-week-old female AKR mice was inoculated with 10^6 SL-2 cells at subcutaneous sites on the back. Three milligrams of purified RI7 208 monoclonal antibody (antimurine transferrin receptor) or monoclonal antibody 19E12 (anti-Thy-1.1) were given on Days 0, 4, and 7. The first injection was intravenous; the succeeding two doses of antibody were intraperitoneal. The figures shown are the mean survival time of mice in each group (89).

The antitumor activity of the antitransferrin receptor antibody TI7 208 was compared to the anti-Thy-1 monoclonal antibody 19E12, previously shown to produce therapeutic effects in the transplantable syngeneic SL-2 leukemia model (87,88). Two major points emerge from this study. One, RI7 208 improved the survival of tumor-bearing mice as much, if not better, than the anti-Thy-1.1 monoclonal antibody. Second, in contrast to the anti-Thy-1 monoclonal antibody 19E12, treatment with the antitransferrin receptor antibody inhibited growth of the primary tumor. Palpable tumors in the antitransferrin receptor antibody-treated mice only became detectable more than 2 weeks after the last injection of monoclonal antibody, implying that the antibody had eliminated 3-4 logs of the initial cell inoculum. At this

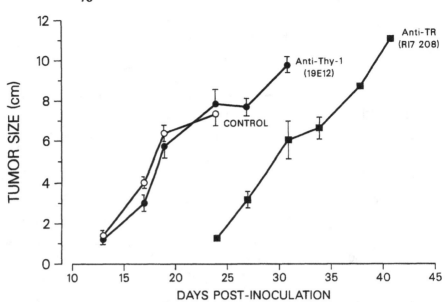

FIGURE 4. The effects of antitransferrin receptor antibody RI7 208 on the growth of SL-2 cells at the primary tumor site in AKR/J mice. The data shown are from the same experiment as shown in Figure 3. Mice were inoculated with SL-2 leukemia cells and given antibodies as described in Figure 3. The figure shows the mean tumor size on each day measured as the average of two perpendicular axes with calipers in each group of mice (89).

time the tumors grew as rapidly in the antibody-treated mice as in the control group. In subsequent experiments in which RI7 208 monoclonal antibody was administered for several weeks, complete inhibition of tumor cell growth in 80% of the mice was obtained. Furthermore, additional experiments have shown that a combination of anti-Thy-1 and antitransferrin receptor antibody in this model system is more effective than either antibody alone.

4. CONCLUDING REMARKS

Antireceptor antibodies directed against growth-related cell surface receptors have antiproliferative effects upon human tumor cells in xenografts and upon transplantable syngeneic murine tumor cells. Whether these antibodies act by blocking receptor function in vivo has not yet been rigorously determined. The antibodies have also provided a means to study hormone-receptor interactions, receptor metabolism, cell type-specific receptor expression, and receptor structure. Much of the basic information which has been obtained regarding receptor distribution, metabolism, and ligand-receptor interactions is useful in evaluating the potential effectiveness of antireceptor antibody therapy. Further, the general observation that proliferating cells express more receptor than quiescent cells was facilitated by having monoclonal antibodies available to probe the cell surface.

Antigen density (or density of bound antibody) may be an important factor in the effectiveness of antireceptor antibody effects on tumor cell proliferation. Therefore, the antiproliferative effects of two or more antireceptor monoclonal antibodies against different receptors present on the same tumor cell surface, or perhaps against different epitopes on the same receptor molecule, would be a worthwhile avenue of investigation. The simultaneous use of two antibodies against two different receptors has additional theoretical appeal, since it provides a novel way to attempt to circumvent the problem of tumor cell heterogeneity. Thus, if a minor cell population in a tumor lacked one receptor in sufficient numbers, but expressed another, it might be possible to prevent its growth with two antireceptor antibodies.

The development of a battery of monoclonal antibodies directed towards growth-related cell surface receptors may provide a new avenue for the treatment of malignant tumors. They will also be used to provide a new means by which to characterize the tumor cell surface and provide information of prognostic value. The utility of monoclonal antibodies against such receptors in cancer therapy should be clarified experimentally within the next few years.

ACKNOWLEDGMENTS

We would like to acknowledge the contributions made by our colleagues to our work cited in this review. From UCSD, Hironubu Sunada, Tomyuki Kawamoto, J. Denry Sato, Gordon Sato, Anh Le, and Gordon Gill; from the Salk Institute, Jane Leslie, Robert Hyman, Ronald Newman, Bishr Omary, Derrick Domingo, and Frederick Lopez.

REFERENCES

1. Flier JS, Kahn CR, Jarrett DB, Roth J. 1976. J Clin Invest 58:1442-1449.
2. Kahn CR, Baird KL, Flier JS, Jarrett DB. 1977. J Clin Invest 60:1094.
3. Appel SH, Anwyl R, McAdams MW, Elias SB. 1977. Proc Natl Acad Sci USA 74:2130.
4. Appel SH, Elias SB, Chauvin P. 1979. Fed Proc 38:2319.
5. Volpe R. 1978. Endocrinol Metab 7:3.
6. Dexhage HA, Bottazzo GF, Bitensky L, Chayen J, Doniach D. 1981. Nature 289:594.
7. Wren S, Haber E. 1977. J Biol Chem 254:6577.
8. Caron MG, Scrinivasan Y, Snyderman R, Lefkowitz RJ. 1979. Proc Natl Acad Sci USA 76:2263.
9. Couraud PO, Delavier-Kutchko C, Curieu-Trautmann O, Strosberg AD. 1981. Biochem Biophys Res Commun 99:1295.
10. Bohnet HG, Shiu RPC, Grinwich D, Friesen HG. Endocrinology 102:1657.
11. Lewin R. 1981. Science 211:38.
12. Haigler HT, Carpenter G. 1980. Biochem. Biophys Acta 598:312.
13. Schreiber AB, Libermann TA, Lax I, Yarden Y, Schlessinger ER. 1983. J Biol Chem 58:846-853.
14. Kawamoto T, Sato JD, Le A, Polikoff J, Sato GH, Mendelsohn J. 1983. Proc Natl Acad Sci USA 80:1337-1341.
15. Masui H, Kawamoto T, Sato JD, Wolf B, Sato G, Mendelsohn J. 1984. Cancer Res 44:1002-1007.
16. Trowbridge IS, Lopez F. 1982. Proc Natl Acad Sci USA 79:1175.
17. Mendelsohn J, Trowbridge I, Castagnola J. 1983. Blood 62:821.
18. Trowbridge IS, Domingo D. 1981. Nature (London) 294:171-173.
19. Barnes D, Sato G. 1980. Cell 22:649-655.
20. Barnes D, Sato G. 1980. Anal. Biochem. 102:255-270.
21. Sato G, Pardee AB, Sirbasku D. 1982. In: Cold Spring Harbor Conferences on Cell Proliferation, Vol 9, Cold Spring Harbor Laboratory, New York.
22. Carpenter G. 1983. Mol Cell Endocrinology 31:1-19.
23. Carpenter G, Cohen S. 1979. Ann Rev Biochem 48:193-216.
24. Schlessinger J, Schreiber BB, Levi A, Lax I, Libermann T, Yarden Y. 1983. In: CRC Critical Reviews in Biochemistry, Vol 14, pp 93-111.
25. Carpenter G. 1981. In: Handbook of Experimental Pharmacology, Vol 57. Tissue Growth Factors (Ed R Baserga), Springer Verlag New York, pp 89-123.

26. Bradshaw R, Ruben JS. 1980. J Supramol Struct 14:183-199.
27. Haigler HT. 1983. In: Growth and Maturation Factors (Ed G Guroff), John Wiley and Sons, New York.
28. Ulrich A, Coussens L, Hayflich JS, et al. 1984. Nature 309:418-425.
29. Lin CR, Chen WS, Kruiger W, et al. 1984. Science 224:843-884.
30. Haigler H, Ash J, Singer SJ, Cohen S. 1978. Proc Natl Acad Sci USA 75:3317-3321.
31. Hunter T. 1984. Nature 311:414-416.
32. Cooper JA, Hunter T. 1981. J Cell Biol 91:878-883.
33. Downward J, Parker P, Waterfield D. 1984. Nature 311:483-485.
34. Cooper JA, Reiss NA, Schwartz RJ, Hunter T. 1983. Nature 302:218-223.
35. Hunter T, Ling N, Cooper JA. 1984. Nature 311:480-483.
36. Merlino GT, Zu Y, Ishii S, et al. 1984. Science 234:417-419.
37. Ushiro H, Cohen S. 1980. J Biol Chem 255:8363-8365.
38. Hunter T, Cooper JA. 1981. Cell 24:741-752.
39. Ek B, Westermark B, Wasteson A, Heldin C-H. 1982. Nature 295:419-420.
40. Kasuga M, Zick Y, Blithe DL, Crettaz M, Kahn CR. 1982. Nature 298:667-669.
41. Roth RA, Cassell DJ. 1983. Science 219:299-301.
42. Roberts AB, Frolik CA, Anzano MA, Sporn MB. 1983. Fed Proc 42:2621-2626.
43. Massague J. 1983. Biol Chem 258:13614-13620.
44. Marquardt H, Hunkapiller MW, Hood LE, et al. 1983. Proc Natl Acad Sci USA 80:4684-4688.
45. Cohen S, Carpenter G, King L Jr. 1980. J Biol Chem 255:4834-4842.
46. Galfre G, Howe SC, Milstein C, Butcher GW, Howard JC. 1977. Nature 266:550-552.
47. Sato JD, Kawamoto T, Le AD, Mendelsohn J, Polokoff J, Sato G. 1984. Mol Biol Med 1:511-529.
48. Gill GN, Kawamoto T, Cochet C, et al. 1984. J Biol Chem 259:7755-7760.
49. Gooi HC, Hounsell EF, Lax I, et al. The carbohydrate specificities of the monoclonal antibodies 29.1, 455 and 3ClB12 raised against the EGF receptor of A431 cells (manuscript submitted).
50. Parker PJ, Young S, Gullich WJ, Mayes EL, Bennett P, Waterfield M. 1984. J Biol Chem 259:9906-9912.
51. Barnes DW. 1982. J Cell Biol 93:1-4.
52. Gill GN, Lazar CS. 1981. Nature 293:305-307.
53. Cowley G, Smith JA, Gusterson B, Hendler F, Ozanne B. 1984. In: Cancer Cells, the Transformed Phenotype (Eds AJ Levine, GF Van deWoude, WC Topp, JD Watson), Cold Spring Harbor Laboratory, New York, pp. 5-10.
54. Hendler FS, Ozanne BW. 1984. J Clin Invest 74:647-651.
55. Steplewski Z, Herlyn D, Maui G, Koprowski H. 1983. Hybridoma 2:1-5.
56. Le A. Unpublished data.
57. Weber W, Bertics PJ, Gill GN. 1984. Immunoaffinity purification of the EGF receptor: stoichiometry of EGF binding of kinetics of self-phosphorylation. J Biol Chem, in press.

58. Jandl JH, Katz JH. 1963. J Clin Invest 42:314-326.
59. Seligman PA, Schleicher RB, Allen RH. 1979. J Biol Chem 254: 9943-9946.
60. Wada HG, Hass PE, Sussman HH. 1979. J Biol Chem 254:12629-12635.
61. Hamilton TA, Wada HG, Sussman HH. 1979. Proc Natl Acad Sci USA 75:6406-6410.
62. Galbraith GMP, Galbraith RM, Faulk WF. 1980. Cell Immunol 49:215-222.
63. Larrick JW, Cresswell P. 1979. J Supramol Struct 11:579-586.
64. Omary MD, Trowbridge IS, Minowada J. 1980. Nature 286:888-891.
65. Judd W, Poodry CA, Strominger JL. 1980. J Exp Med 152:1430-1435.
66. Haynes BF, Hemler M, Cotner T, et al. 1981. J Immunol 127:347-351.
67. Trowbridge IS, Omary MB. 1981. Proc Natl Acad Sci USA 78: 3030-3043.
68. Sutherland R, Delia D, Schneider C, Newman R, Kemshead J, Greaves M. 1981. Proc Natl Acad Sci USA 78:4515-4519.
69. Goding JW, Burns GF. 1981. J Immunol 127:1256-1258.
70. Omary MB, Trowbridge IS. 1981. J Biol Chem 256:12888-12892.
71. Scheider C, Sutherland R, Newman RA, Greaves MF. 1982. J Biol Chem 257:8516-8522.
72. Trowbridge IS, Lesley J, Schulte, R. 1982. J Cell Physiol 112:4903-4910.
73. Klausner RD, Ashwell G, van Renswoude J, Harford JB, Bridges KR. 1983. Proc Natl Acad Sci USA 80:2263-2266.
74. Dautry-Varast A, Ciechanover A, Lodish HF. 1983. Proc Natl Acad Sci USA 80:2258-2262.
75. Bleil JD, Bretscher MS. 1982. EMBO J 1:351-355.
76. Bretscher MS. 1983. Proc Natl Acad Sci USA 80:454-458.
77. Hopkins CR, Trowbridge IS. 1983. J Cell Biol 97:508-521.
78. Faulk WP, Hsi B-L, Steven PL. 1980. Lancet ii:309-392.
79. Shindelman JE, Ortmeyer AE, Sussman HH. 1981. Int J Cancer 27:329-334.
80. Gatter KC, Brown G, Trowbridge IS, Woolston RE, Mason DY. 1983. J Clin Pathol 36:539-545.
81. Habeshaw JA, Bailey D, Stansfeld AG, Greaves MF. 1983. Br J Cancer 47:327-351.
82. Habeshaw JA, Lister TA, Stansfeld AG, Greaves MF. 1983. Lancet i:498-500.
83. Kvaloy S, Langholm R, Kaalhus O, et al. 1984. Int J Cancer 33:173-177.
84. Lesley J, Domingo D, Schulte R, Trowbridge I. 1984. Exp Cell Res 150:400-407.
85. Trowbridge IS, Lopez F. 1982. Proc Natl Acad Sci USA 79: 1175-1179.
86. Trowbridge IS, Lesley J, Schulte R. 1982. J Cell Physiol 112:403-410.
87. Bernstein ID, Nowinski RC. 1982. In: Hybridomas in Cancer Diagnosis and Treatment (Eds MS Mitchell, HF Oettgen), Raven Press, New York, pp 97-112.
88. Bernstein ID, Tam MR, Nowinski RC. 1980. Science 207:68-71.

89. Trowbridge IS, Newman RA, Domingo DL, Sauvage C. 1984. Biochem Pharmacol <u>33</u>:925-932.
90. Trowbridge IS, Newman RA. 1984. <u>In</u>: Monoclonal Antibodies to Receptors: Probes for Receptor Structure and Function (Ed MF Greaves), Chapman and Hall, London, pp 237-261.

4. MONOCLONAL ANTIBODY THERAPY FOR PATIENTS WITH LEUKEMIA AND LYMPHOMA*

KENNETH A. FOON, ROBERT W. SCHROFF and PAUL A. BUNN

1. INTRODUCTION

Monoclonal antibodies are extremely useful in the classifi-cation of leukemia and lymphoma (1) and there is considerable interest in the utilization of monoclonal antibodies for treat-ment as well (2-4). A number of studies utilizing monoclonal antibodies for the treatment of leukemia and lymphoma in animal tumor models (5) and humans (6-17) have recently been reported. These studies have emphasized the pharmacokinetics of monoclonal antibody therapy, toxicity, biodistribution, and responses to these murine-derived antibodies (Table 1).

2. CLINICAL RESPONSES

The responses in patients with B-cell derived lymphoma (6), T-cell chronic lymphocytic leukemia (T-CLL) (7), cutaneous T-cell lymphoma (CTCL) (8,9,11,13,14), B-cell chronic lymphocytic leu-kemia (B-CLL) (10-13,15), acute lymphoblastic leukemia (ALL) (3,16), and acute myelogenous leukemia (AML) (17) treated with a variety of antibodies were very transient. In most cases, there was a 50%-75% drop in the circulating leukemia cell count, which returned to the baseline level within 24-48 hr following the antibody infusion. The typical "sawtoothed" pattern reported by numerous investigators is shown for a B-CLL patient treated with T101 in Figure 1 (12). Patients with cutaneous T-cell lymphoma

*This project has been funded at least in part with Federal funds from the Department of Health and Human Services under contract number NO1-CO-12910 with Program Resources, Inc. The contents of the publication do not necessarily reflect the views or policies of the Department of Health and Human Services, nor does mention of trade names, commercial products, or organi-zations imply endorsement by the U. S. Government.

Table 1. Monoclonal antibody clinical trials for lymphoma and leukemia.

Disease	Antibody/Class	Specificity	No. of patients	Toxicity	Effect	Institution	Reference
B-CLL	T101/IgG$_{2a}$	T65	13	Dyspnea, hypotension, fever (101-102°F)	Transient reduction in circulating cells	NCI	12,13
B-CLL	T101/IgG$_{2a}$	T65	4	Dyspnea, hypotension, fever, malaise, urticaria	Transient reduction in circulating cells	Univ. Calif. San Diego	10,11
B-CLL	IgG$_{2b}$ and IgG$_1$	Idiotype	1	Fever, urticaria	Transient reduction in circulating cells	NCI	15
B-lymphoma	Ab89/IgG$_{2a}$	Lymphoma	1	Renal (transient)	Transient reduction in circulating cells	Dana-Farber	6
B-lymphoma	4D6/IgG$_{2b}$	Idiotype	1	None	Complete remission 36+ months	Stanford	20
B-lymphoma	IgG$_1$ or IgG$_{2a}$ or IgG$_{2b}$	Idiotype	7	Fever, chills, nausea, dyspnea, rash, diarrhea	4 of 7 partial remissions	Stanford	21
CTCL	T101/IgG$_{2a}$	T65	12	Dyspnea, fever, (101-102°F)	Minor remission 4 patients	NCI	13,14
CTCL	L17F12/IgG$_{2a}$	Leu-1	6	Dyspnea, hives, cutaneous pain	Minor remission 5 of 7 patients	Stanford	8,9
CTCL	T101/IgG$_{2a}$	T65	4	Fever, chills, malaise, bronchospasm, urticaria	Minor remissions	Univ. Calif. San Diego	11
T-CLL	L17F12 (anti-Leu-1)/IgG$_{2a}$	Leu-1	1	Renal, hepatic (transient)	Transient reduction in circulating cells	Stanford	7
T-ALL	L17F12/IgG$_{2a}$ 12E7/IgG$_1$ 4H9/IgG$_{2a}$	Leu-1 T & B cells T cells	8	Sporadic coagulopathy	Transient reduction in circulating cells	Stanford	3
ALL	J5/IgG$_{2a}$	CALLA	4	Fever (101-102°F)	Transient reduction in circulating cells	Dana-Farber	16
AML	PM/81/IgM AML-2-23/IgG$_{2b}$ PMN 29/IgM		3	Urticaria, fever, back pain, arthralgia, myalgia	Transient reduction in circulating cells	Dartmouth	17

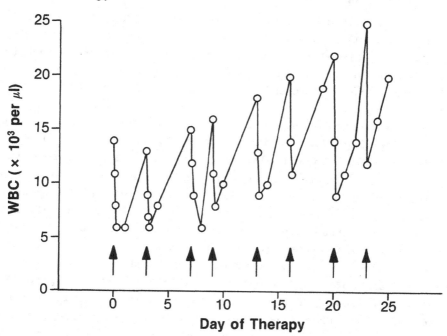

FIGURE 1. Response of circulating leukemia cells to infusion of
T101. Arrows represent infusion of 50 mg of antibody. The solid
line represents the absolute number of white blood cells (WBC)
per microliter.

were treated with either the T101 or anti-Leu-1 antibodies that
recognize the same 65,000- to 67,000-dalton glycoprotein antigen
(18,19). Improvement in cutaneous lesions was demonstrated in
approximately one half of these patients; however, these responses did not persist for more than a few weeks beyond the cessation of antibody therapy. Clearly, with the possible exception
of anti-idiotype antibodies (20,21) (described below), unconjugated antibodies will rarely, if ever, have an important therapeutic role for patients with leukemia and lymphoma. These
early trials, however, have generated critical information for
future trials with drugs and toxins conjugated to monoclonal
antibodies.

3. IN VIVO ANTIBODY LOCALIZATION AND ANTIGENIC MODULATION

Dose-dependent in vivo localization was demonstrated by flow cytometry on circulating bone marrow, lymph node, and cutaneous tumor cells in all of the reported studies. This was an issue of in-depth investigation in our own studies using the T101 murine IgG$_{2a}$ antibody.

We studied the number of circulating leukemia cells that labeled in vivo with varying doses of T101. To assess in vivo binding of T101 to circulating leukemia cells, fluorescein-labeled goat antimouse immunoglobulin was added in vitro directly to the cells without supplying additional T101 in vitro. In this way, only cells that bound with T101 in the circulation following an intravenous infusion of T101 would label as positive. Positive results were obtained in all patients and are shown in the lower curve in Figure 2. Immediately following a 1-mg infusion of T101, circulating cells demonstrated up to 25% staining; following a 10-mg infusion, circulating cells were up to 60% stained. From 25%-80% of circulating cells were stained in vivo with either rapid or prolonged infusions of 50 and 100 mg of T101 antibody.

To determine the maximum ability of cells removed from T101-treated patients to label with T101, excess T101 antibody was added to cells in vitro followed by fluorescein-labeled goat antimouse IgG antiserum (upper curve of Fig. 2). In actuality, this procedure permits detection of both in vivo and in vitro bound T101, although we simply use the term "in vitro" here for clarity. This curve was compared with a curve of the same cells at the identical time point following infusion of T101, which were treated with the fluorescein-labeled goat antimouse antiserum only. In this way we could determine the number and intensity of cells staining with T101 in vivo and compare this with the same cells treated with excess T101 in vitro. The difference between these curves was due to the T65 antigen not bound in vivo. Figure 2 shows a comparison of in vivo (lower curve) versus in vitro staining (upper curve) for one representative patient from each treatment group. At 1 mg, a small proportion of circulating cells was stained in vivo (25%) while excess antibody

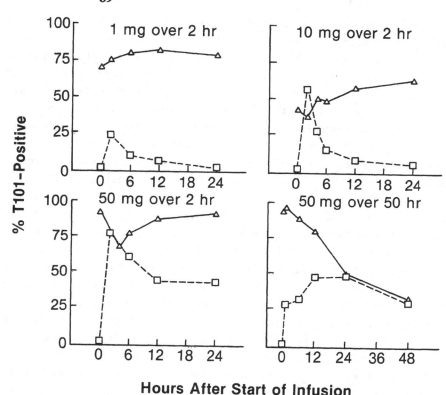

FIGURE 2. In vivo versus in vitro binding of antibody by circulating B-CLL cells. The lower curve (□) represents in vivo
labeling of circulating leukemia cells with T101 antibody.
The upper curve (△) represents the same circulating leukemia
cells treated in vitro with excess T101 and then labeled with
fluorescein-tagged goat antimurine antibody. The difference
between these curves at each time point measured represents
the number of cells that were not labeled in vivo with T101.

stained 80% of the cells in vitro. Immediately following a 2-hr
infusion of 10 mg of antibody, there was a maximum number of in
vivo stained circulating cells, which equaled the number stained
in vitro. This declined over the next few hours, either because
T101 was lost from the cell surface membrane or because these
cells were removed from the circulation. Following a rapid infusion of the 50-mg dose of T101 (actually 40 mg, as the infusion
was discontinued due to pulmonary toxicity), there was again

maximum in vivo binding of T101 of circulating cells immediately following therapy. However, when 50 mg of T101 was added over a prolonged infusion (1 mg/hr), the in vivo and in vitro binding did not coincide until 24 hr after the initiation of therapy, and at that time only about 50% of the circulating cells expressed the T65 antigen, most likely due to antigenic modulation (21).

Bone marrow samples were obtained to determine in vivo localization of T101 antibody in leukemic bone marrow cells. As indicated in Figure 3, bone marrow cells were removed prior to infusion, as well as 2 and 24 hr following infusion of 10 mg of T101 antibody. Prior to therapy, 90% of the cells stained in vitro with T101 antibody. Eighty-one percent of the leukemic bone marrow cells were labeled in vivo 2 hr after infusion of T101, with only 10% additional cells labeled when excess T101 was added in vitro. When excess antibody was added in vitro to the 2-hr specimen, staining was less intense than when excess antibody was added to the sample taken prior to therapy (Fig. 3) (compare dotted lines, top and middle curves), indicating a decrease in T65 antigen density most likely due to antigenic modulation. Twenty-four hours after therapy, the bone marrow cells no longer had in vivo bound T101 on the cell surface membrane and the cells had fully recovered expression of the T65 antigen.

In contrast to the results obtained following 10-mg infusions over 2 hr, prolonged infusions of 20–100 mg of T101 monoclonal antibody (1–2 mg/hr) resulted in less in vivo binding to the cell surface membranes of circulating and bone marrow cells for patients with B-CLL and CTCL. By 5 hr into the infusion, no greater than 15% of the cells demonstrated in vivo binding, and at the end of 12 hr virtually no in vivo binding was observed. This was due to nearly 100% modulation of T65 antigen secondary to this prolonged infusion. Furthermore, while T65 antigen expression declined, the expression of B-cell antigens (B1, BA1) and immunoglobulin remained unchanged in patients with B-CLL, and other T-cell antigens such as Leu-4 (pan-T) and Leu-3 (T-helper) remained unchanged in patients with CTCL. An example of this can be found in Figure 4, where maximum staining with

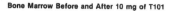

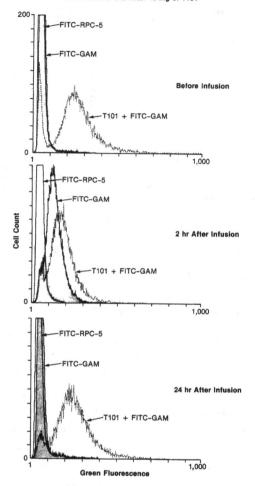

FIGURE 3. In vivo labeling of bone marrow cells with T101 antibody. Bone marrow cells were taken from the same patient before infusion of a 10-mg dose of monoclonal antibody, 2 hr after this infusion of 10 mg of T101, and 24 hr after infusion. The solid line represents staining with fluorescein isothiocyanate (FITC)-conjugated RPC-5 as a negative control. The shaded area represents in vivo bound T101 antibody identified by incubating the cells with FITC-conjugated goat antimouse (GAM) antiserum. The dotted line represents the same leukemia bone marrow cells treated in vitro with excess T101 prior to the addition of the FITC-conjugated GAM antiserum.

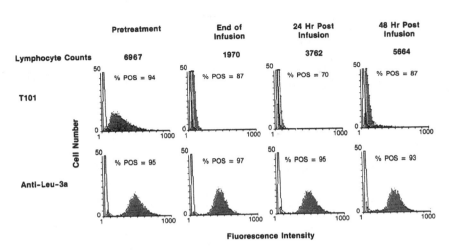

FIGURE 4. Flow cytometry curves for a patient with cutaneous T-cell lymphoma and Sézary cell leukemia treated with 50 mg of T101 over 12 hr. Cells were stained <u>in vitro</u> with excess T101 or anti-Leu-3a antibodies. Note the loss of the T65 antigen at the 2-, 24-, and 48-hr post-treatment time points, with no change in expression of the Leu-3a antigen.

both T101 and anti-Leu-3a is shown. As the total number of circulating Sézary cells is reduced to approximately one third following the T101 infusion, the intensity of T101 staining is reduced dramatically. Even as the circulating Sézary cells return to the pretreatment numbers, the intensity of staining is still reduced due to antigenic modulation. In the lower set of curves, the expression of the Leu-3a antigen remains unchanged, demonstrating that only the T65 antigen is modulated by T101. This clearly demonstrated that antigenic modulation is highly specific for only the antigen identified by the antibody used for therapy.

4. REGENERATION OF T65 SURFACE ANTIGEN

To assess the ability of leukemic cells that had undergone near total loss of T65 antigen to regenerate this antigen, <u>in vitro</u> studies were performed (22). Circulating leukemic cells as well as bone marrow cells were obtained both before treatment and at the end of a 50-hr infusion in a patient receiving a

50-mg dose. Cells were cultured in the presence or absence of 10 g/ml of T101. Cells were harvested at 0, 1, 2, 3, 4, and 7 days and were assessed for T65 antigen expression. In the absence of T101 in cultures, bone marrow tumor cells that had lost the T65 cell surface antigen in vivo (4% T101 positive) reexpressed the T65 antigen to pretreatment levels (79% T101 positive) by 4 days, whereas identical specimens in the presence of T101 remained negative. Conversely, specimens taken before therapy lost the T65 antigen in vitro in the presence of T101 (2% T101 positive), whereas the same specimens in the absence of T101 underwent increases in T65 antigen density and actually became greater than 80% T101 positive, a phenomenon that we have previously observed (unpublished observations). Similar findings were observed with circulating leukemic cells. These experiments confirm that in vivo loss of the T65 antigen after 50-hr infusions is a reversible phenomenon. Furthermore, these experiments indicate that the loss of T65 antigen by CLL cells can be reproduced in vitro and persists for periods of up to 7 days in the presence of T101. Similar results have been reported using J5 antibody, which recognizes the common acute lymphoblastic leukemia antigen (CALLA) (23).

5. FATE OF T65 ANTIGEN AND BOUND T101 ANTIBODY

To assess the fate of cellular bound antibody, in vitro studies were performed by using ^{125}I-labeled T101 (21). Leukemic cells obtained from B-CLL patients before therapy were cultured in the presence of 0.1 μg/ml ^{125}I-labeled T101 under conditions known to induce modulation of the T65 antigen of CLL and normal lymphoid cells (24). After culture, the cells were washed, the amount of cell-associated ^{125}I-T101 was determined by gamma counting, and the specimens were trypsinized to determine the percentage of cell-associated ^{125}I-T101 that was exposed to the cell surface as opposed to intracellular exposure. Replicate specimens were processed for immunofluorescence after the initial period of culture. Optimal binding of the radiolabeled T101 to the B-CLL cells occurred within 30 min, and no appreciable decline in the amount of cell-associated radiolabel occurred during the initial 8 hr of culture. On the contrary, decreases in cell surface T65 antigen density, as measured by immunofluorescence staining, occurred within 15 min of initiating the culture, and approximately 50% of the cell surface antigen was undetectable after 8 hr of culture. The trypsinization studies indicated that the majority of the cell-bound ^{125}I-T101 was originally trypsin sensitive on the cell surface. Over the initial 8 hr of culture, the majority of the radiolabeled T101 became trypsin insensitive, suggesting intracellular accumulation of the label. By the end of the 24-hr culture, most of what little radiolabel remained was again trypsin sensitive. These findings are consistent with rapid internalization of the radiolabeled T101 during the first 8 hr of culture, followed by release of the radiolabeled antibody from the cells during the subsequent 16 hr. This may be a more generalized phenomenon of lymphoid-associated antigens, as internalization of CALLA has also been described (23).

6. THERAPEUTIC APPLICATIONS OF ANTIGENIC MODULATION: IMMUNOCONJUGATES

Antigenic modulation might be used to therapeutic advantage, particularly in a system in which there is rapid internalization of the antibody such as is found with T101. As described in Chapter 1, numerous investigators are evaluating immunoconjugates of monoclonal antibodies coupled to toxins, drugs, and radioisotopes in animal models. A review of antibodies coupled to isotopes for human studies is presented in Chapter 7. The data in animal models clearly demonstrate a far greater efficacy of antibody conjugated to toxins than unconjugated free antibody (25,26). Many of these toxic substances, such as ricin, diphtheria, and abrin toxins, contain subunits that mediate binding to the target cells and independent subunits responsible for the toxic mechanism. In most cases, only the toxic subunit is coupled to the monoclonal antibody, and binding to the target cell is mediated through specific interaction of antibody to the appropriate antigen. In this situation, the ability of an antibody to induce antigenic modulation and internalization of

the antibody-antigen complex may facilitate access of the drug
or other toxic substance to its site of action within the cell
and therefore augment the effectiveness of immunoconjugate therapy. The data presented in this study indicate that modulation
of the T65 antigen is accompanied by internalization of antigen-
antibody complexes and suggest that treatment of B-CLL and CTCL
cells with T101 immunoconjugates under conditions that bring
about rapid and extensive modulation of the T65 antigen may
provide an effective means of therapy. Our future clinical
trials will address the role of immunoconjugates with drugs
such as doxorubicin and vindesine and toxins such as the A chain
of ricin and gelonin in the treatment of B-CLL and CTCL. We are
currently studying [111]indium conjugated to T101 for imaging
CTCL and B-CLL patients. Lesions as small as 0.5 cm have been
detected (27).

7. TOXICITY WITH UNCONJUGATED ANTIBODIES

The only major predictable complication witnessed in the
NCI clinical trial with T101 was shortness of breath and chest
tightness either during or immediately following the 2-hr
infusion of T101 at dosages of 50 mg or greater (12-14). Similar
toxicity was reported by Dillman and co-workers also with the
T101 antibody (10,11) and with anti-idiotype antibody therapy
in patients with circulating lymphoma cells (21). While this
toxicity was transient and had no residual side effects, patients
were extremely uncomfortable, and we were forced to stop therapy
in all of the patients who experienced dyspnea. Chest x-rays
and lung scans were normal in all of the patients except one
whose lung scan showed a perfusion abnormality and another
whose chest x-ray showed a pulmonary infiltrate. These abnormal
findings resolved within 1 to 2 weeks. We therefore hypothesized
that the rapid infusion of large quantities of monoclonal antibody, bound to circulating leukemia cells and/or normal T
lymphocytes, led to leukoagglutination. The agglutinated cells
were then removed in the pulmonary microcirculation, causing
pulmonary emboli and infarctions. There was no evidence that
this pulmonary toxicity was caused by an anaphylactic reaction,

as there was no response to epinephrine and measurable IgE levels were not demonstrated (see Chapter 6). Furthermore, some patients were subsequently treated with prolonged infusions of the same antibody without recurrence of these symptoms. Patients treated with rapid infusions (1-2 hr) of much greater dosages of the 9.2.27 antimelanoma monoclonal antibody (500 mg), which does not bind to any circulating cells, never developed this toxicity. We have completely eliminated this toxicity with T101 by infusing the antibody at rates of 1-2 mg/hr.

Rare patients have developed hypotension and tachycardia following the infusion of murine monoclonal antibody (10,12). This complication was most likely anaphylactic and responded to administration of fluid and epinephrine. Therapy was stopped in all of the patients who developed this complication. Urticaria, also an anaphylactic immediate hypersensitivity reaction, was quite common and rapidly responded to antihistamines. Patients developing urticaria were pretreated with antihistamines prior to subsequent treatment. Fever, chills, flushing, nausea, and vomiting have been reported but have generally been minor problems. Occasional patients have developed a transient reduction in their creatinine clearance and an elevation of their liver enzymes, probably due to immune complexes between the murine monoclonal antibody and circulating free antigen (6, 7).

8. ANTI-IDIOTYPE MONOCLONAL ANTIBODY

A more specific approach to the use of monoclonal antibody therapy is the use of anti-idiotype monoclonal antibodies. Immunoglobulin molecules have a unique region in their variable portion, termed the "idiotype." The idiotype for every immunoglobulin molecule is different. Since B-cell diseases are clonal, each tumor cell expresses the same immunoglobulin molecule; therefore, the idiotype is theoretically identical on every tumor cell. In this unique situation, the idiotype is therefore a tumor-specific antigen.

A group of investigators from Stanford developed a monoclonal antibody to the idiotypic determinant from a patient with a B-cell lymphoma who had become resistant to cytotoxic drugs and interferon (28). This patient was treated with 8 doses of anti-idiotype monoclonal antibody i.v. in a dose-escalation fashion and he eventually entered a complete remission that has persisted for over 3 yr (20,21). Seven additional patients have been treated, with only 4 partial remissions lasting from 1 to 6 months (21). The mechanism of the antitumor activity of anti-idiotype antibodies is not known. One possibility is that anti-idiotypes have a direct antitumor effect. A likely additional factor is the activation of host effector mechanisms and the augmentation of an antitumor process already present in the host.

Our first patient treated with an anti-idiotype monoclonal antibody at the NCI was a patient with B-CLL and bulky lymph-adenopathy. He was treated sequentially with an IgG_{2b} antibody to a total dose of 1 g and then an IgG_1 antibody to a total dose of 750 mg (15). There was no response because circulating idiotype (50 µg/ml) prevented binding of antibody to tumor cells. Although we were able to reduce the circulating idiotype level by 75% with plasmapheresis, we were still unable to iden-tify murine antibody on circulating tumor cells.

A number of problems regarding anti-idiotype therapy must be addressed. Developing murine anti-idiotype antibodies is a labor-intensive project and is not practical on a large scale. It is hoped that this process can be refined as new technology is developed. In addition, anti-idiotype antibodies in our studies have been patient-specific and therefore can be used to treat only a single patient. It has recently been reported that some tumors are biclonal. This problem was identified using anti-idiotype antibodies and immunoglobulin gene rearrangement studies (29,30). One approach to identifying patients with more than one clone prior to developing the anti-idiotype antibody would be to perform immunoglobulin gene rearrangement studies on all patients under consideration. If more than one clone is identified, then the patient would either not be a candidate for anti-idiotype therapy, or more than one antibody would have to be developed for that patient. Finally, it has been demon-strated that some tumors have unstable idiotypes likely due to genetic mutation (31).

9. PURGING OF AUTOLOGOUS BONE MARROW WITH MONOCLONAL ANTIBODIES

Another attractive therapeutic approach using monoclonal antibodies is to "clean up" autologous bone marrow prior to bone marrow transplantation (Fig. 5). Patients with acute lymphoblastic leukemia have had bone marrow removed and treated with the J5 monoclonal antibody (anti-CALLA) and complement to selectively deplete the tumor cells (32). Following bone marrow removal, treatment, and storage, patients were treated with high-dose chemotherapy and radiation therapy and then "rescued" with their J5 antibody-treated autologous bone marrow. A similar approach to therapy has been described using the pan-B reacting anti-B1 monoclonal antibody to clean up autologous bone marrow from patients with non-Hodgkin's lymphoma (33). All of the lymphoma patients treated achieved a complete remission and had stable bone marrow engraftment by 8 wk. There was no major acute or chronic toxicity; B cells were detected by 2 months after transplantation and normal immunoglobulin levels were

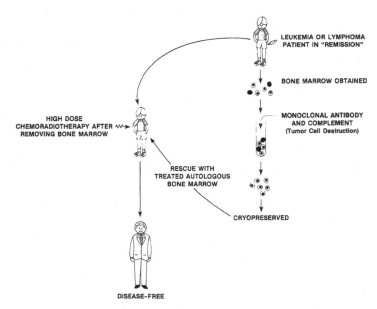

FIGURE 5. Schema for monoclonal antibody treatment of bone marrow for autologous bone marrow transplantation.

demonstrated by 6 months. Six of 8 patients were disease-free
in unmaintained remission from 3-20 months after transplantation. The results of these trials are preliminary but have
clearly demonstrated that antibody-treated autologous bone
marrow is capable of restoring hematopoiesis. Long-term results
will be necessary to determine whether these therapies have
been successful.

10. CONCLUSION

The use of monoclonal antibody and antibody immunoconjugates
in the treatment and radioimaging of leukemia and lymphoma is
in its infancy. While much work needs to be done to clarify
many of the issues surrounding the use of monoclonal antibodies,
it has been clearly demonstrated in both animal tumor models and
humans that antibody alone and antibody conjugates can be safely
administered with minor adverse reactions and, in selected
cases, have been shown to have therapeutic effects. Problems
such as nonspecific localization of antibody in the reticuloendothelial system, host antibody responses, and antigenic
heterogeneity are all major obstacles to safe and effective
therapy with monoclonal antibodies. While anti-idiotype antibodies are highly specific and have demonstrated remarkable
responses in a small number of patients, problems such as
biclonality of some lymphomas, instability of the idiotype,
and the difficulty in making "tailor-made" antibodies for
individual patients clearly limit the role for anti-idiotype
therapy. Purging of bone marrow with antibodies and complement
(or coupled to toxins) is limited to only a few diseases.
However, in some studies, investigators have removed tumor
cells in vitro from the bone marrow, the bone marrow has
engrafted, and a number of patients have been rendered disease-
free for over 1 yr. This may prove to be an important application of monoclonal antibody therapy and warrants further studies.
This therapy, of course, bypasses most of the problems associated
with intravenous infusion of monoclonal antibodies described
above. Perhaps the most important future role for monoclonal
antibody therapy will be in patients with minimal disease in

the "adjuvant" setting, where antibody conjugates may localize and destroy micrometastatic deposits of tumor cells. We remain cautiously optimistic in exploring these exciting new approaches to cancer therapy.

REFERENCES

1. Foon KA, Schroff RW, Gale RP. 1982. Blood 60:1-19.
2. Ritz J, Schlossman SF. 1982. Blood 59:1-11.
3. Levy R, Miller RA. 1983. Fed Proc 42:2650-2756.
4. Oldham RK. 1983. J Clin Oncol 1:582-590.
5. Foon KA, Bernhard MI, Oldham RK. 1982. J Biol Resp Modif 1:277-304.
6. Nadler LM, Stashenko P, Hardy R, et al. 1980. Cancer Res 40:3147.
7. Miller RA, Maloney DG, McKillop J, Levy R. 1981. Blood 58:86-87.
8. Miller RA, Levy R. 1981. Lancet 2:226-230.
9. Miller RA, Oseroff AR, Stratte PT, Levy R. 1983. Blood 62:988-995.
10. Dillman RO, Shawler DL, Sobol RE, et al. 1982. Blood 59:1036-1045.
11. Dillman RO, Shawler DL, Dillman JB, Royston I. 1984. J Clin Oncol 2:881-890.
12. Foon KA, Schroff RW, Bunn PA, et al. 1984. Blood 64:1085-1094.
13. Foon KA, Schroff RW, Sherwin SA, Oldham RK, Bunn PA, Hsu S-M. 1983. In: Monoclonal Antibodies and Cancer (Eds BD Boss, RE Langman, IS Trowbridge, R Dulbecco), Academic Press, New York, pp 39-52.
14. Bunn PA, Foon KA, Schroff RW, et al. 1983. Blood 62 (suppl 1):210a (abstract).
15. Giardina SL, Schroff RW, Kipps TJ, et al. 1985. J Immunol, in press.
16. Ritz J, Pesando JM, Sallan SE, et al. 1981. Blood 58:141-152.
17. Ball ED, Bernier GM, Cornwell GG, McIntyre OR, O'Donnell JF, Fanger MW. 1983. Blood 62:1203-1210.
18. Royston I, Majda JA, Baird SM, Meserve BL, Griffiths JC. 1890. J Immunol 125:725-731.
19. Martin PT, Hansen JA, Siadak AW, Nowinski RC. 1981. J Immunol 127:1920-1923.
20. Miller RA, Maloney DG, Warnke R, Levy R. 1982. N Engl J Med 306:517-522.
21. Lowder JN, Meeker TC, Maloney DG, Thielmans K, Miller RA, Levy R. 1984. Proc Am Soc Clin Oncol 3:250.
22. Schroff RW, Farrell MM, Klein RA, Oldham RK, Foon KA. 1984. J Immunol 133:1641-1648.
23. Pesando JM, Ritz J, Lazarus H, Tomaselli KJ, Schlossman SF. 1981. J Immunol 126:540-544.
24. Schroff RW, Klein RA, Farrell MM, Stevenson HC. 1984. J Immunol 133:2270-2277.

25. Bernhard MI, Foon KA, Oeltmann TN, et al. 1983. Cancer Res 43:4420-4428.
26. Hwang KM, Foon KA, Cheung PH, Pearson JW, Oldham RK. 1984. Cancer Res 44:4578-4586.
27. Bunn PA, Carrasquillo JA, Keenan AM, et al. 1984. Lancet ii(8413):1219-1221.
28. Hatzubai A, Maloney DG, Warnke R, Levy R. 1981. J Immunol 126:2397-2402.
29. Sklar J, Cleary ML, Thielemans K, Gralow J, Warnke R, Levy R. 1984. N Engl J Med 311:20-27.
30. Giardina SL, Schroff RW, Woodhouse CS, et al. 1985. Blood, in press.
31. Raffeld M, Cossman J. 1984. Blood 64 (Suppl. 1):183a (abstract).
32. Ritz J, Bast RC, Clavell LA, et al. 1982. Lancet 2:60-63.
33. Nadler LM, Takvorian T, Botnick L, et al. 1984. Lancet 2:427-431.

5. MONOCLONAL ANTIBODY THERAPY OF SOLID TUMORS

PAUL G. ABRAMS and ROBERT K. OLDHAM

1. INTRODUCTION

Sufficient preclinical and clinical data are now available on the use of monoclonal antibodies (MoAb) in the treatment of human solid tumors to describe their likely role in the treatment of cancer (1). The initial trials focused on the usual phase I considerations of toxicity and tolerance, but added the localization of the antibody in tumor deposits and the distribution of antibody in normal and neoplastic tissues as concurrent investigations (2-4). There is now a considerable body of evidence from the administration of 1 mg to several grams of a number of murine monoclonal antibodies that these agents are well tolerated by patients. Although clinical responses to unconjugated antibody have generally not been striking, there is unequivocal evidence that antibody binds to individual tumor cells after intravenous injection (5).

Although biodistribution studies utilizing antibody conjugated to isotopes have demonstrated that a considerable amount of antibody also traffics to the liver, spleen, and other organs of the reticuloendothelial system (6), the antibody/isotope conjugates are retained selectively in the tumor considerably longer than in normal tissues where binding may be nonspecific.

These findings support the strategy of diagnosing, staging, and treating human malignancies with monoclonal antibodies conjugated to isotopes, drugs, and toxins. Several reviews have been written on the use of monoclonal antibody in the treatment of human solid tumors that include historical data concerning the use of heteroantisera and other antibody preparations in cancer treatment (1,7-9). The purpose of this chapter will be

K.A. Foon and A.C. Morgan, Jr. (eds.), *Monoclonal Antibody Therapy of Human Cancer.* Copyright © 1985. Martinus Nijhoff Publishing, Boston. All rights reserved.

to assess critically more recent data available on the use of unconjugated antibody in the treatment of human solid tumors to provide some perspective on the potential clinical uses of unconjugated antibody and a basis for designing therapies with antibody conjugated to drugs, isotopes, and toxins.

2. DEVELOPMENT OF MONOCLONAL ANTIBODIES FOR THERAPY

A number of different murine monoclonal antibodies have been developed that may be assessed in clinical trials in patients with solid tumors (10). For cancers such as melanoma, lung, breast, and colon cancer, more than ten antibodies for each have been described and characterized. No doubt there will be a large variety of new monoclonal antibodies both of murine derivation and, eventually, from human sources available in the future. It is apparent, therefore, that the limitation for the use of monoclonal antibody preparations as clinical reagents will not be due to a shortage of antibody preparations (1). Although the ideal antibody (i.e., _absolute_ specificity for cell surface antigens for a particular tumor) has not been identified for human solid tumors, a number have sufficient selectivity to warrant clinical testing.

Criteria to select monoclonal antibodies appropriate for clinical trials will depend upon the ultimate projected role of the antibody in diagnosis or treatment of the particular disease. A "Special Tracks" retreat sponsored by the Biological Response Modifiers Program of the National Cancer Institute in 1983 was unable to reach a consensus on the criteria to select or reject an antibody for clinical trials. Nonetheless, it seems reasonable to us to consider the following "rebuttable presumptions*" favoring a particular antibody for _in vivo_ application.

1. Antibody binds to an antigen on the cell surface;
2. Antibody binds with high affinity;
3. Antigen highly expressed on cell surface and found on most or, preferably, all cells in a tumor;

---

*i.e., antibodies that meet these criteria have a presumption in their favor as clinical agents; those that do not have a burden of showing why they are nonetheless desirable.

4. Antigen expressed at very low levels on a very limited number of normal tissues and/or found only on occasional cells in normal tissues;
5. Antigen-antibody complexes internalize[†];
6. Antibody mediates antibody-dependent cellular cytotoxicity (ADCC)[‡];
7. Biodistribution studies reveal negligible uptake of antibody by the reticuloendothelial system (RES).[†]

Antibodies that satisfy all these criteria are more likely to have clinical utility than those that do not, but it is important to recognize that most of these judgments are relative. Thus, one antibody is preferred (presumptively) over others if it binds to more rather than less tumor cells, with higher rather than weaker affinity, where each cell expresses greater rather than lesser surface antigen, etc. Thus, a familiarity with prior experience in the field, with attention to these criteria, will help determine whether a given antibody, not previously tested in clinical trials, appears promising. In addition, there may be reasons why certain antibodies that bind to few cells could be of clinical interest if it could be shown, for example, that it binds to "stem cells" but not necessarily to more differentiated cells that lack the potential for unlimited growth. According to this scheme, however, the "burden of proof" is on an antibody that does not meet these criteria to show it is nonetheless worthy of clinical interest.

The antibody, whether conjugated or not, presumably must reach the tumor bed to be effective. Smaller antibodies (IgG rather than IgM) or antibody fragments may be more likely to diffuse from the vascular compartment out into the tumor bed. Our studies indicate that the greater the amount of whole IgG antibody infused into the vascular compartment, the more antibody is delivered to the tumor cell bed (5). We have even demonstrated that doses of 200-500 mg of antibody can saturate all sites on the tumor cell in cutaneous melanoma metastases.

[†]Especially important for some immunoconjugates (toxins and drugs).

[‡]Most important for unconjugated antibody, but may also increase the potency of conjugates.

While access to the tumor is clearly critical, however, retention within that tumor bed may be equally or more important. Thus, antibody fragments may diffuse more quickly into the tumor nodule, but whole antibody may be retained for a longer period of time within that same nodule. It is not clear which factors are more important and this will most likely depend on the ultimate use of the antibody as a targeting vehicle. At this time the paramount issue is developing methods to study these different antibodies in clinical trials.

3. USE OF UNCONJUGATED ANTIBODIES IN CLINICAL TRIALS

There are certain important principles in the design and execution of clinical trials using monoclonal antibodies for the treatment of patients with solid tumors (1), and a competent laboratory must be able to monitor the fate and distribution of antibody in clinical trials (see Table 1). To demonstrate that antibody reached the tumor cells themselves and bound to antigen in vivo, for example, biopsy specimens obtained subsequent to infusion of antibody must be tested by immunohistochemistry techniques on frozen specimens and/or flow cytometry on cell suspensions (5,11,12). Immunohistochemistry indicates the distribution of antibody within the tumor nodule in contrast to the surrounding normal tissues; flow cytometry allows accurate quantitative assessment of the percentage of cells binding antibody and of the degree of "saturation" (number of sites bound/total number of sites available). Additional monitoring should include quantitating circulating antibody (pharmacokinetics), measuring circulating antigen, if such exists, determining the presence of immune complexes, and antiglobulin and anti-idiotypic responses to murine antibody. The latter responses will be especially critical in determining the dose and timing constraints of conjugate therapy; significant levels of either may also alter biodistribution of the infused antibody. Finally, careful clinical observations should be made in the course of monoclonal antibody studies in patients.

Table 1. Critical parameters in phase I trials of monoclonal antibodies in patients with cancer.

A. Pre-therapy

   1. Tumor sample for antigen expression
   2. Serum for circulating antigen

B. During and/or after therapy

   1. Antibody localization: Immunohistochemistry on fresh frozen tumor sample
   2. Antigenic saturation: Flow cytometry on fresh tumor cell suspension
   3. Pharmacokinetics
   4. Immune complexes
   5. Antiglobulin and/or anti-idiotype responses (May need to follow for months)

It is clear then that these antibodies, being biologic substances, require both laboratory and clinical expertise to carry out meaningful investigations. These preparations should not be considered as just another class of drugs to be given by individuals or groups expert in the use of chemotherapy. Biological substances have clinical and biological activities very different from the chemicals used in chemotherapy. The immune system already has receptors and/or mechanisms for dealing with biologic substances that do not exist for chemical compounds that are not normally part of human biology.

4. CLINICAL TRIALS

At the Biological Response Modifiers Program, National Cancer Institute, a series of melanoma patients was treated with the 9.2.27 IgG$_{2a}$ murine monoclonal antibody developed by Morgan and co-workers (13). This antibody recognizes a 250 kd glycoprotein/proteoglycan antigen on the surface of melanoma cells. It binds to >90% melanomas freshly removed from patients, exhibits both high affinity and quantitatively high binding to melanomas, and does not appear to bind to normal tissues with the exception of occasional basal cells, blood vessel endothelium, and sebaceous glands in the skin. It met most of the criteria discussed earlier and, therefore, appeared to be an excellent candidate antibody for early clinical trials. After intravenous administration of antibody, we used flow cytometry to determine the percentage of cells that bound antibody and the degree of saturation of antigenic binding sites by in vivo antibody. We used immunohistochemistry on frozen sections of freshly removed nodules to determine the distribution of administered antibody in the tumor. As shown in Table 2, we could show antibody staining tumor cells at doses above 10 mg, with a definite trend to greater staining with higher doses. At the 10 mg and 1 mg doses, we generally did not detect antibody in the tumor by these techniques. The immunoperoxidase studies indicated that areas of tumor most accessible to blood vessels or lymphatic spaces stained first at the 50 mg level and only with higher doses did the other cells bind detectable antibody (Fig. 1).

The flow cytometry studies indicated that, starting at doses of 200 mg and higher, first binding to all tumor cells and then saturation of all available binding sites on the tumors could be achieved. The latter finding is important for several reasons:

(i) It defines the maximum useful dose for a single injection;

(ii) It determines the dose range expected for immunoconjugate delivery;

(iii) It ensures that maximum doses of immunoconjugate reach every cell decreasing the chances of selecting resistant cells due to suboptimal delivery; and

(iv) It ensures that hypoxic cells, those furthest from blood vessel access, receive the maximum deliverable dose.

Pharmacokinetic parameters were measured that defined the peak antibody concentration and the half-life of the antibody in these studies. Peak level and half-life were affected by anti-globulin levels and trace labeled antibody preparations were very useful in making these measurements. There were no antitumor responses.

Table 2. In vitro* and in vivo† reactivity of 9.2.27 antibody with melanoma cells in cutaneous skin lesions.

Patient	Dose 9.2.27	Days Post treatment	9.2.27 reactivity			
			Flow cytometry (%) % positive cells		Immunoperoxidase‡ score	
			In vitro	In vivo	In vitro	In vivo
A.F.	Pretreatment		80	ND§	++	–
	1 mg	1	92	0	++	–
D.F.	Pretreatment		83	ND	++	–
	1 mg	1	0	0	+	–
	50 mg	1	72	0	++	+
	200 mg	1	ND	ND	++	+
M.F.	Pretreatment		97	ND	++	+
	10 mg	1	98	2	+	–
	100 mg	1	72	50	+	+
	200 mg	4	98	91	+	+
B.C.	Pretreatment		90	ND	++	+
	200 mg	1	73	71	+	–
C.S.	Pretreatment		76	ND	++	–
	1 mg	1	91	0	++	+
	200 mg	1	41	35	+	–
A.T.	Pretreatment		0	ND	++	–
	50 mg	1	ND	ND	++	+
	200 mg	1	14	50	++	–
M.G.	Pretreatment		76	1	++	++
	50 mg	4	97	1	++	++
J.S.	Pretreatment		ND	ND	++	–
	50 mg	1	ND	ND	++	+
	100 mg	1	ND	ND	++	++

*In vitro reactivity refers to reactivity when excess 9.2.27 was added during the staining procedure.
†In vivo reactivity refers to endogenously bound 9.2.27 after i.v. antibody therapy.
‡Staining of melanoma cells with 9.2.27 was graded on a + to ++ scale which represents a combination of both percent positive cells and intensity of staining.
§ND, not done.

109

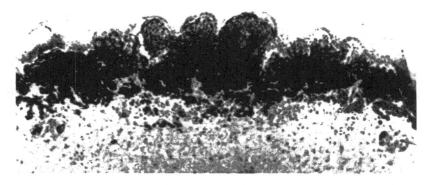

9.2.27 In Vitro

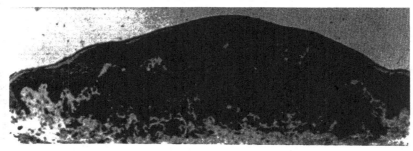

Post 50 mg 9.2.27

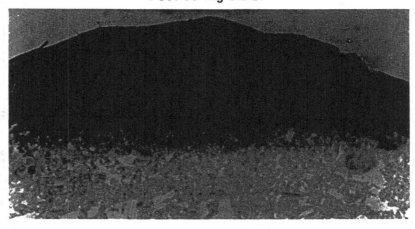

Post 100 mg 9.2.27

FIGURE 1. Distribution of 9.2.27 in melanoma tumor nodule as a function of dose. Top figure shows in vitro saturation with 9.2.27 and the lower figures are in vivo localization after 50 and 100 mg doses.

It was then important to determine where besides the tumor nodules the antibody localized. Radioimmunolocalization using 9.2.27 conjugated to indium-111 was done to study the biodistribution of the antibody. As shown in Figure 2, labeled antibody does go to the reticuloendothelial system as well as to tumor. The hepatic uptake was especially significant, but studies with ^{131}I-labeled 9.2.27 by another group have shown much less in that organ (Ø. Fodstad, personal communication). This difference may be more apparent than real. At this time the most likely explanation is that hepatic halogenases remove ^{131}I and it then gets "excreted" from cells as iodide, whereas the free ^{111}In is protein bound and remains in liver cells. These studies raise critical issues concerning the relevance of unlabeled antibody studies to conjugates since the material conjugated and the effect of the conjugation procedure on the antibody may profoundly influence the biodistribution.

Phase I studies have also been performed with antibody to a 97 Kd antigen (p97) on the surface of melanomas and other tumors. Studies have also been done with antibody 48.7 directed at the same antigen recognized by 9.2.27 (11). These studies confirmed the results discussed above. Houghton and co-workers have shown major tumor regressions in 3 of 12 patients with melanoma using a monoclonal antibody that binds to the disialoganglioside G_{D3} and is lytic with human complement and mediates ADCC (14). Tumor biopsies during and after treatment demonstrated lymphocyte and mast cell infiltration, mast cell degranulation, and complement deposition.

Larson and co-workers have gone one step further and administered an anti-p97 antibody labeled with therapeutic doses of ^{131}I to show therapeutic activity for isotope conjugates in patients with melanoma. Localization of the labeled antibody has been seen and evidence of minor tumor regression was noted (15). Thus, these early clinical trials have progressed rapidly from antibody alone to therapeutic attempts with labeled antibody. Recently, an antimelanoma antibody/toxin conjugate has been approved for phase I clinical trials. All of these studies, taken

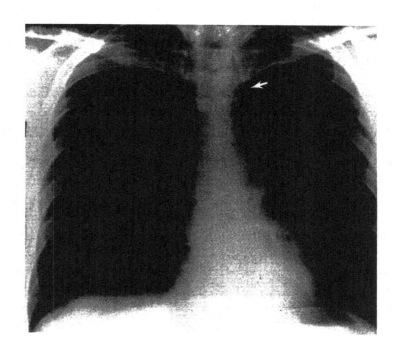

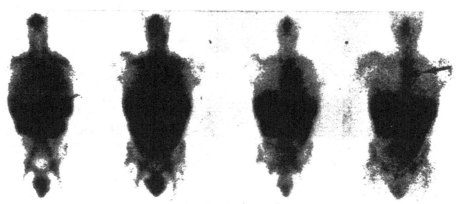

FIGURE 2. A. Chest x-ray with arrow pointing to a hilar lesion. B. 9.2.27-¹¹¹In radioimaging with arrow pointing to the same hilar lesion seen on chest x-ray.

together, demonstrate the feasibility of the immunoconjugate approach and will no doubt lead to future trials that will begin to demonstrate efficacy (16).

The other major solid tumor system studied with in vivo monoclonal antibody has been gastrointestinal malignancies. Sears and co-workers treated more than 20 patients with gastrointestinal malignancies with antibody 17-1A (IgG_{2a}) and demonstrated localization of the antibody in the tumor (4,12). From 15-1000 mg per patient have been given as single doses without severe side effects. Circulating immunoglobulin has been seen for as long as 50 days compared to 9.2.27 which has a half-life of approximately 30 hours and disappears from the serum within days and certainly by 1 week. This may be due to the low affinity of 17-1A and its shedding from the tumor cell surface. In addition, 17-1A has a much wider normal tissue reactivity than 9.2.27 and thus the "sink" for antibody deposition and subsequent shedding is much larger. These issues have not, however, been directly addressed.

Antiglobulin responses to 17-1A appeared to be dependent on the dose of antibody. Only one patient receiving doses above 366 mg produced antimouse immunoglobulin whereas the majority of those treated with lower doses had definite evidence of these responses. They reported but did not definitely document clinical antitumor responses in three of these patients, and postulated that this salutory effect may be due to antibody-macrophage interactions within the tumor bed. On the other hand, they have attempted to correlate these clinical responses with development of anti-idiotype antibodies to 17-1A, but have not documented that nonresponders did not develop anti-idiotypes. They suggested that a combination of high doses of antibody to reduce the antiglobulin response and the use of an IgG_{2a} subclass might be a reasonable approach in studying further patients with unconjugated antibody with gastrointestinal carcinoma.

Dillman and co-workers have given infusions of anti-CEA monoclonal antibody to several patients with evidence of clinical localization without antitumor response (17). A brief report on the use of an IgG_3 monoclonal antibody which had in vitro cytotoxicity against human gastrointestinal carcinoma was reported by Lemkin and co-workers in abstract form (18). Eight patients were treated with infusion of this antibody preparation over several days. Complement consumption and fever were noted and murine antiglobulins appeared to give a syndrome consistent with mild serum sickness. Immunohistologic evidence of antibody localization was seen but no clinical responses were observed.

An interesting report on the use of human heterologous antibody produced by Melino and co-workers from London appeared recently in abstract form (19). Antibodies were produced by allogeneic immunization in 12 volunteers. These antibodies were used to target daunorubicin and chlorambucil in 12 neuroblastoma patients over the age of 2. These preparations were well tolerated and no antiglobulin, allergic, or toxic effects were noted. Marked antitumor responses were reported in 9 of 12 patients and all patients are said to be disease-free after more than 3 years. Careful analysis of a complete report on these findings will be necessary before conclusions can be drawn.

A summary of recent serotherapy trials using monoclonal antibody for solid tumors is shown in Table 3. No attempt has been made to summarize the older data with heteroantisera as this has been recently reviewed (8). More recent reports with rabbit, goat, and even human allogeneic sera are receiving some attention, but have not been summarized here. While these approaches may be of value and are of interest, they would seem to lack the essential features of reproducibility, high titer, unlimited quantity, and molecular purity needed to proceed with large-scale clinical trials. Emerging evidence on the use of antibodies derived by in vitro or in vivo immunization of humans for the purpose of producing human monoclonal antibody are of interest, but no clinical trials have been carried out with human monoclonal antibodies. These preparations possess certain advantages but may also have certain inherent disadvantages as reviewed earlier (1). The use of conjugated preparations in vitro and in animal tumor models is discussed elsewhere in this book. With respect to monoclonal antibody serotherapy trials certain conclusions can be summarized (Table 4).

Table 3. Monoclonal antibody serotherapy trials
in patients with solid tumors.

Institution	Disease	MoAb	References
U. of Penn. (Wistar)	GI cancer	17-1A	(4,12)
UCLA	GI cancer	CCOLI	(18)
U. Calif. San Diego	Colon cancer	065	(17)
U. Calif. San Diego	Melanoma	Ab to p97 Ab to p240	(3)
Fred Hutchinson Cancer Center	Melanoma	Ab to p97	(15)
Swedish Hosp. Med. Center, Seattle	Melanoma	48.7 and Ab to p97	(11)
National Cancer Institute	Melanoma	9.2.27	(5)
Sloan-Kettering, New York City	Melanoma	Anti-GD3	(14)

Table 4. Summary - Monoclonal antibody serotherapy trials.

1. Intravenous murine-derived MoAb can be given safely by prolonged infusion (> 1 hr) without immediate side effects.
2. Bronchospasm and hypotension have followed rapid infusion (5 mg/hr) with antibodies that bind to circulating cells.
3. Antigenic modulation occurs following treatment with some MoAbs but not all MoAbs.
4. Free antigen may be detected in the serum following MoAb treatment.
5. Clear evidence of selective localization of infused antibody in solid tumors is available.
6. Antibodies to mouse cells may develop following MoAb therapy.
7. There is considerable variation with respect to toxicity, bioavailability, and activity related to immunoglobulin class, antigen, and distribution to tumor.

Many studies are in progress with antibody conjugates in vitro and in nu/nu mouse human xenograft tumor models (20), some showing excellent toxicity in vitro and in vivo for human tumor cells. Large numbers of phase I studies should be initiated with antibody conjugates in man in the very near future.

5. FUTURE APPLICATIONS IN MAN AND PROSPECTIVES

The information available from these early trials suggests certain principles for optimal therapy with monoclonal antibodies that may be important in the design of future studies (Table 5). These factors should all be considered at either the preclinical or early clinical stages so that investigators can adequately interpret the results of trials.

Table 5. Optimization of monoclonal antibody therapy.

Antibody Specificity

    Immunoperoxidase
    Radiolocalization

Antigen Characterization

    Biochemical nature
    Topography
    Epitope (different parts of the antigen molecule)
    Heterogeneity

Antibody-Antigen Interaction

    Turnover of antibody bound to tumor cells
    Degree of antibody internalization
    Antigen levels in serum

Antibody Delivery

    Dose
    Regimen
    Route
    Pharmacokinetics
    Comparison of various agents conjugated
      to same antibody

The monoclonal antibodies used to date have been of murine origin and are thus foreign proteins in man. Other factors that could provoke toxicity other than reaction to an infused foreign protein include circulating antigen that may form immune complexes and the syndromes associated with them such as serum sickness, or the presence of antigen on circulating cells that has been noted to provoke severe bronchospasm and skin rash without other associated allergic symptoms. The likely explanation for the latter is leukoagglutination and/or release of vasoactive substances in small bronchial arterioles (21). The toxicities of monoclonal antibody therapy are listed in Table 6. Recognition of the problems and their causes has led to strategies to ameliorate these toxicities (21), thereby enhancing the potential therapeutic activity of these preparations.

Based on the information available at this time, unconjugated antibodies are not likely to have an important therapeutic use. As reviewed elsewhere in this book, minor clinical effects with unconjugated antibody have been seen mainly in leukemia and certain lymphomas. In the area of solid tumors, only the report of Houghton and co-workers on possible clinical effects of unconjugated anti-GD3 antibody in melanoma is encouraging (14). The major conclusions to be drawn from these studies in solid tumors are that monoclonal antibodies are safe, target to tumor, and that strategies can be designed to bind to all available antigenic sites on all tumor cells.

Table 6. Clinical toxicity in monoclonal antibody trials.

Fever	Dyspnea
Chills	Hypotension/tachycardia
Flushing	Anaphylactic/anaphylactoid reactions
Urticaria	Serum sickness
Rash	Increased creatinine
Nausea/vomiting	Headache
Bronchospasm*	

*Pulmonary toxicity (dyspnea, bronchospasm, etc.) has been observed with monoclonal antibodies that bind to circulating cells.

The in vitro selectivity and activity, as well as some pre-
clinical in vivo activity without toxicity in animals, achieved
with immunoconjugates are encouraging, although a great deal more
basic research needs to be done. Very early studies with the use
of immunoconjugates of antibody and isotopes in human solid
tumors have shown encouraging localization and even some evidence of therapeutic effects (15). These data, together with
historical data on the use of heteroantisera, drug, and isotope
conjugates suggest that immunoconjugates are likely to be very
useful in improving the selectivity and efficacy of cancer
treatments in the near future (22-25).

It is worth commenting on the likely ultimate outcome of this
area of research. All of our current data suggest antibody will
traffic to the reticuloendothelial system so that even the most
highly specific antibody by in vitro assessment will exhibit
substantial in vivo normal organ distribution. Thus, the immunoconjugates will most likely improve the therapeutic index (tumor
response vs. toxicity) by targeting toxic agents directly to
tumor and decreasing, but not eliminating, normal organ exposure.
If this, rather than an elusive search for absolute tumor specificity in vivo, is accepted as an appropriate goal, then immunoconjugates with monoclonal antibodies should have a rapid and
wide acceptance in the armamentarium of weapons against cancer.
The lack of selectivity of systemic chemotherapy means that any
substantial improvement in the selective delivery of toxic
substances to tumor cells through monoclonal antibody technology
will be a step in the right direction.

One factor that could potentially dampen this enthusiasm is
the known heterogeneity of cancer and the ability of cancer
cells to mutate. If one uses a single antibody or a combination
of a few antibodies that together bind only to a portion of the
tumor cells, or if the small percentage of the true replicating
cell (stem cell) is not eliminated, eventual recurrence of the
tumor, perhaps with resistant cells, will result. It seems
logical, therefore, to "type" human tumors with a panel of
antibodies and to deliver toxic substances utilizing "cocktails"
of antibodies sufficient to bind strongly to all the tumor

cells for each patient. This approach requires a considerable amount of testing for each patient and a "typing" of one or more tumors from each patient.

Such approaches may be much more custom-tailored than is easily approachable through the product development paradigm that has been used with some success in the development of new cancer drugs. Clinical investigators have heretofore been satisfied with statistical analysis of empirically selected therapies. Indeed, many reputations have been built because a particular alphabet of anticancer drugs actually worked in certain diseases. Immunoconjugates place added burdens on investigators: selecting correct combinations for individual patients and explaining the 20%, 40%, or 80% of nonresponses on the basis of biology, not statistics.

REFERENCES

1. Oldham RK. 1983. J Clin Oncol 1:582-590.
2. Larson SM, Brown JP, Wright PW, et al. 1983. J Nucl Med 24:123-129.
3. Sobol RE, Dillman RO, Smith JD. 1981. In: Hybridomas in Cancer Diagnosis and Treatment (Eds MS Mitchell, HF Oettgen), Raven Press, New York, pp 199-206.
4. Sears HF, Mattis J, Herlyn D, et al. 1982. Lancet 1:762-765.
5. Oldham RK, Foon KA, Morgan AC, et al. 1984. J Clin Oncol 2:1235-1242.
6. Goldenberg DM, DeLand FH. 1982. J Biol Resp Modif 1:121-136.
7. Foon KA, Bernhard MI, Oldham RK. 1983. J Biol Resp Modif 1:277-304.
8. Rosenberg SA, Terry WD. 1977. Adv Cancer Res 25:323-388.
9. Dillman R. 1984. Monoclonal Antibodies in the Treatment of Cancer. CRC Critical Reviews in Oncology/Hematology 1:357-385.
10. Boss BD, Langman RE, Trowbridge IS, Dulbecco R (Eds). 1983. Monoclonal Antibodies and Cancer. Academic Press, New York.
11. Goodman GE, Beaumier P, Hellstrom I, Fernyhough B, Hellstrom KE. 1985. J Clin Oncol 3:340-352.
12. Sears HF, Herlyn D, Steplewski Z, Koprowski H. 1984. J Biol Resp Modif 3:138-150.
13. Morgan AC Jr, Galloway DR, Reisfeld RA. 1981. Hybridoma 1:27-36.
14. Houghton AN, Mintzer D, Cardon-Cardo C, et al. 1985. Proc Natl Acad Sci USA 82:1242-1246.
15. Larson SM, Carrasquillo JA, Krohn KA. 1982. In: Proceedings of the Third World Congress of Nuclear Medicine and Biology, vol 4. Pergamon Press, New York, pp 3666-3669.

16. Morgan AC Jr, Pavanasassivam G, Hwang KM. 1984. In: Protides of the Biological Fluids (Ed H Peeters), Pergamon Press, New York, pp 773-777.
17. Dillman RO, Beauregard JC, Shawler DL, et al. 1983. In: Protides of the Biological Fluids (Ed H Peeters), Pergamon Press, New York, pp 353-358.
18. Lemkin S, Tokita K, Sherman G, et al. 1984. Proc Am Soc Clin Oncol 3:47.
19. Melino G, Elliott P, Cooke KB, et al. 1984. Proc Am Soc Clin Oncol 3:47.
20. Oldham RK. 1984. Cancer Treat Rep 68:221-232.
21. Foon KA, Schroff RW, Bunn PA, et al. 1984. Blood 64:1085-1094.
22. Key ME, Bernhard MI, Hoyer LC, et al. 1983. J Immunol 139:1451-1457.
23. Bernhard MI, Foon KA, Oeltmann TN, et al. 1983. Cancer Res 43:4420-4428.
24. Bernhard MI, Hwang KM, Foon KA, et al. 1983. Cancer Res 43:4429-4433.
25. Hwang KM, Foon KA, Cheung PH, et al. 1985. Cancer Res 44:4578-4586.

6. HUMAN IMMUNE RESPONSES TO MURINE MONOCLONAL ANTIBODIES

ROBERT W. SCHROFF and HENRY C. STEVENSON

1. INTRODUCTION

Monoclonal antibodies have great potential for the diagnosis, staging, and therapy of human tumors. As reviewed in the preceding chapters, over a dozen different monoclonal antibodies have been employed for the treatment of advanced malignant diseases since the first clinical trial was reported in 1980 (1). Since all of the monoclonal antibodies utilized to date have been derived from mice, it was expected that perhaps certain hypersensitivity reactions to xenogeneic proteins might occur when they were injected into humans, as was found in earlier clinical trials with crude heterologous antisera (2). While the experiences of investigators in this field are still too limited to provide exact estimates of the frequency of hypersensitivity reactions to monoclonal antibodies, it does not appear that these types of immune responses will pose insurmountable obstacles to the clinical use of monoclonal antibodies. Information is now being acquired on hypersensitivity reactions to murine monoclonal antibodies in humans, and it is this subject which will be reviewed in this chapter.

There are four major types of hypersensitivity reactions, any of which could be encountered with monoclonal antibody infusions. The acquisition of information on the types of reactions one may encounter with monoclonal antibody therapy is ongoing, and the mechanisms involved in those reactions are still being determined. However, it would seem appropriate to at least attempt to classify these reactions with respect to the four accepted types of hypersensitivities. We will begin with a brief review of the current accepted mechanisms of action of these four types of hypersensitivity reactions.

K.A. Foon and A.C. Morgan, Jr. (eds.), *Monoclonal Antibody Therapy of Human Cancer.* Copyright © 1985. Martinus Nijhoff Publishing, Boston. All rights reserved.

Type I reactions represent the classical allergic-type response to a foreign antigen. Typically, this consists of allergic-type conjunctivitis, rhinitis, or urticaria in its mildest forms, asthma in its intermediate form, and anaphylaxis (hives, asthma, and hypotension chiefly) in its most severe form. The mechanism of action of this hypersensitivity reaction is based upon the secretion of IgE in response to a foreign antigen. These IgE molecules are preferentially bound by Fc receptors on mast cells throughout the body, sensitizing the mast cell for degranulation when exposed to foreign antigens. The chemical mediators released by the mast cells following degranulation are felt to be responsible for the vast majority of symptoms observed in type I hypersensitivity reactions.

Type II hypersensitivity reactions are characterized by the induction of an IgG response to a foreign antigen. Ordinarily, this humoral response is responsible for the clearance of foreign antigens and does not produce adverse symptoms except under two circumstances: (1) the production of IgG that not only binds the foreign antigen but also cross-reacts with "self" antigens in normal tissues, or (2) the production of IgG which becomes incorporated into circulating immune complexes. Symptoms from type II reactions are related to any specific tissue injury that might occur, or the symptoms of immune complex disease (below) should they occur.

Type III hypersensitivity reactions are characterized by the formation of circulating immune complexes. These immune complexes can be trapped within the capillary beds of the body and activate the complement cascade. Normal tissues in the region of immune complex deposition may be damaged; immune complex diseases can present as a symptom complex consisting of painful joints, fever, and a variable degree of urticaria within 8 to 24 hours after infusion of the foreign antigen. Other forms of immune complex disease include certain vasculitic syndromes (as observed in hepatitis antigen-associated vasculitis) and immune complex-mediated chronic glomerulonephritis.

Type IV hypersensitivity reactions are felt to be mediated by antigen-specific T lymphocytes which migrate to the site of foreign antigen deposition and promote a local cellular reaction. Examples of type IV reactions include the tuberculin skin test reaction and poison ivy rash, both of which appear 48 to 72 hours after challenge with an antigen.

Precise understanding of the mechanisms involved in many of the clinical responses to complications of monoclonal antibody administration is very limited at present. However, as a framework for the discussion of these responses, we have attempted to relate each response to one of the four accepted types of hypersensitivity reactions.

2. ALLERGIC (TYPE I)-MEDIATED REACTIONS OBSERVED FOLLOWING MONOCLONAL ANTIBODY INFUSIONS

Since monoclonal antibodies are murine-derived proteins, it seems reasonable that in addition to being recognized as antigens in the human host, they might act as allergens in patients who are predisposed to atopic clinical manifestations. However, clear-cut allergic reactions to monoclonal antibody infusions have not been reported. This may stem from a variety of facts, including the low number of patients treated with monoclonal antibodies to date. However, there has been a substantial number of patients with atopic histories who have received monoclonal antibody infusions. Despite allergic symptoms to environmental antigens and drugs such as penicillin, these patients have not demonstrated allergic reactions to monoclonal antibody infusion. Immunoglobulin preparations may not be allergenic per se since infusions of human gamma globulin (as immunoglobulin replacement) does predispose hypogammaglobulinemic patients to IgE-mediated reactions. Infusions of horse antiserum preparations did produce a low incidence of allergic-type reactions in transplant patients, but these were not clearly related to the production of IgE and could be explained by other mechanisms (3). It is also possible that murine immunoglobulin might be a more potent stimulator of blocking antibodies (IgG) than of IgE. One monoclonal antibody which has seemingly induced allergic-type reactions is the T101 antibody. This monoclonal antibody identifies an antigen found on normal and malignant human T lymphocytes and is also found on certain malignant B lymphocytes (including B-cell chronic lymphocytic leukemia, CLL) (4). Following administration of the T101 monoclonal antibody in patients with T- and B-cell malignancies, a number of significant and severe allergic-type reactions have been noted by ourselves (5,6) and by others (7). These reactions include the development of urticaria, pulmonary bronchospastic reactions, and combinations of hives, bronchospasm, and hypotension (reviewed in Chapter 4). In our experience, these symptoms can develop as early as 15 minutes following the infusion of the T101 monoclonal antibody and are usually reversible by administration of antihistamines with or without the addition of adrenalin. This form of pulmonary toxicity can be experienced during the initial antibody treatment and is highly dependent upon the rate of antibody infusion. This toxicity is likely related to the antibody causing cellular microaggregates in the circulation which are cleared by the pulmonary microvasculature, as is addressed in Chapter 4 (5,6).

The development of hives or urticaria has not been restricted to use of the T101 antibody, but has been reported in clinical trials of other antibodies as well (5-10,12). In a trial of gastrointestinal tumors with the 17-1A monoclonal antibody (10), urticaria in two patients was associated with previous histories of urticaria in response to stress. Similar predisposing factors have not been noted in our experience, or in other trials in which urticaria was observed. Similarly, anecdotal reports of bronchospasm in association with either elevated IgE levels (7) or associated with a host antimurine immunoglobulin response (11) have appeared in the literature, but have not been confirmed by subsequent reports (10). The observations to date suggest that the clinical symptoms observed may be due to immune complex formation between antibody and circulating cells with subsequent pulmonary deposition, and that the mechanism involved may more closely resemble that of a type III hypersensitivity reaction.

In an attempt to better define the etiology of the clinical reactions observed following T101 administration, several tests were performed. Skin testing revealed that virtually 100% of patients, regardless of their atopic history (most patients treated with T101 were not atopic), developed positive skin tests to intradermal challenge with the T101 monoclonal antibody within 15 minutes. In contrast, melanoma patients tested by intradermal inoculation with the antimelanoma antibody 9.2.27 and a lymphoma patient tested with an anti-idiotype antibody (both of which were IgG_{2a} antibodies like T101) had negative skin tests (Table 1). No evidence of an IgE-mediated mechanism for this immediate skin test hypersensitivity response to T101 could be demonstrated, including attempts to transfer T101 skin test reactivity to monkeys by Prausnitz-Kustner testing, demonstrate elevated serum or urinary histamine levels, demonstrate elevated total T101 specific IgE levels, or demonstrate binding of T101 to basophils in vitro (Stevenson et al., unpublished observations). Similarly, experiments designed to determine whether T101 binds directly to basophils and triggers degranulation were negative. Thus, it is possible that the administration of the T101 monoclonal antibody, in a high percentage

Table 1. Skin test reactivity to murine monoclonal antibody (MoAb) preparations of patients entering MoAb therapy trials at the NCI.

| Antibody | Disease | No. of Patients | Mean diameter of erythema/induration at indicated time following skin test | |
			15 min	24-48 hr
T101	CTCL	6	18.8 mm	0
T101	CLL	2	20.2 mm	0
9.2.27	Melanoma	6	0	0
Anti-idiotype	Lymphoma	1	0	0

CTCL: cutaneous T-cell lymphoma
CLL: chronic lymphocytic leukemia

of patients, will indirectly cause mast cell degranulation, presumably by binding of antibody to circulating T101 antigen-positive lymphoid cells and deposition in capillary beds or the interstitial space.

3. GENERATION OF IgG ANTIBODY (TYPE II)-MEDIATED REACTIONS FOLLOWING MONOCLONAL ANTIBODY INFUSIONS

One of the primary concerns in the clinical use of murine monoclonal antibodies has been the development of host anti-murine antiglobulin. This type of antibody response could potentially result in the formation of anti-idiotypic antibody capable of inhibiting the localization of murine antibody on the tumor cells (blocking antibody), and/or the formation of immune complexes with subsequent immune complex-mediated tissue damage (type III hypersensitivity reactions).

Table 2 illustrates the frequency of anti-murine antibody responses in clinical trials where such a response was evaluated. Several important points can be drawn from the studies performed to date. First, the response rates appear to be dependent on the disease group being treated. None of the patients with chronic lymphocytic leukemia (CLL) developed an antiglobulin response to infusion of the T101 antibody, while a majority of the patients with cutaneous T-cell lymphoma (CTCL) did develop a response to the same antibody. In disease groups such as melanoma, only a portion of the population developed an anti-globulin response. In CLL patients, the inability to develop an antiglobulin response probably relates to the hypogamma-globulinemic state of these patients. Our studies have indicated, however, that this hyporesponsiveness is not simply a reflection of low serum immunoglobulin levels in these patients, in that pretreatment serum immunoglobulin levels were approximately one quarter that of healthy controls, while pretreatment antiglobulin levels were only one tenth of those detected in the control population (13).

Table 2. Frequency of host antimurine immunoglobulin responses in phase I trials of monoclonal antibodies.

Institution	Disease	Antibody	Class	No. of responders/ total no. of patients	Reference
NCI	CLL	T101	IgG2a	0/11	5,13
UCSD	CLL	T101	IgG2a	0/4	7
NCI	CTCL	T101	IgG2a	4/4	13,14
UCSD	CTCL	T101	IgG2a	2/4	7
Stanford	CTCL	Anti-Leu-1	IgG2a	4/7	8
NCI	ATL	Anti-Tac	IgG2a	0/1	16
Stanford	ATL	Anti-Leu-1	IgG2a	1/1	17
NCI	B lymphoma	Anti-idiotype	IgG2a & IgG1	0/1	18
Stanford	B lymphoma	Anti-idiotype	IgG1, IgG2a, IgG2b	5/9	19,20
Dartmouth	AML	PM-81, 29 & 6 AML-2-23	IgM	1/4	9
Wistar Institute	GI tumors	17-1A	IgG2b	9/18	10
NCI	Melanoma	9.2.27	IgG2a	3/9	13,21
Univ. of Wash.	Melanoma	8.2, 96.5, 48.7 whole Ig	IgG1 & IgG2a	7/9	12
		Fab		8/17	12

UCSD: Univ. of California, San Diego; ATL: adult T-cell leukemia; AML: acute myelogenous leukemia

The data generated in clinical trials to date indicate that antiglobulin response rates do not appear to be determined by the isotype of the infused antibody. In addition to whole antibody molecules, murine Fab and $F(ab')_2$ fragments have also been demonstrated to be immunogenic in man (12). Sears and co-workers (10) have suggested that the initial dose of antibody administered may play a role in determining whether an antibody response ensues. Of colon cancer patients treated with a single dose of the 17-1A antibody (reactive with colon cancer cells), 8 of 9 patients receiving 200 mg doses or less of antibody developed antiglobulin responses, while 8 of 9 patients receiving greater than 200 mg doses failed to develop a response. While several patients receiving total doses of greater than 200 mg have demonstrated anti-mouse antibody responses, at the National Cancer Institute and elsewhere, the multiple-dose design of these trials has not made it possible to confirm this apparent development of tolerance with a single high dose of antibody.

Of primary interest have been the class and specificity of the antiglobulin response in man. The experiences of investigators who have evaluated the specificity of host antimurine immunoglobulin responses are summarized in Table 3. In most cases, the human antibody response has been cross-reactive with most or all mouse immunoglobulin classes. In several cases, a small proportion of the patients' responses, or a small component of a given patient's response, has been specific for the administered antibody (anti-idiotypic). In these cases, the development of an anti-idiotypic antiglobulin response would appear to be evidence that the host antiglobulin response is a primary immune response (assuming that the individual has never before encountered this particular antigen) that is directed against the unique antigen-binding site of the administered antibody. Alternatively, such an anti-idiotypic response could result if the idiotype of the murine antibody cross-reacted with an idiotype to which that individual had been exposed previously. Such a cross-reactive idiotype need not even be from the same species (15). It is not at all clear that the nonidiotypic component of the antiglobulin response in patients

Table 3. Class and specificity of host antimurine immunoglobulin responses.

Institution	Disease	Antibody	Class of responding human antibody	Specificity	Reference
NCI	CTCL	T101	Predominantly IgG	All murine IgG isotypes	13,14
NCI	Melanoma	9.2.27	Predominantly IgG	All murine IgG isotypes, isotypes, significant anti-idiotypic component in 1 patient	13,21
Dartmouth	AML	PM-81, 29 & 6	Predominantly IgG	Murine IgM, but not IgG	9
Stanford	CTCL	Anti-Leu-1	Not described	Murine IgG and IgM, minor anti-idiotypic component	17
Stanford	ATL	Anti-Leu-1	Predominantly IgM	Not determined	8
Wistar Institute	GI tumors	17-1A	Not described	Partially anti-idiotypic	10

receiving monoclonal antibody therapy is likewise the result of primary sensitization with a never-before-seen antigen. Investigators at Stanford (8), as well as ourselves (13), have reported host antimouse antiglobulin responses which are reactive with mouse IgG isotypes other than that of the infused antibody. Similarly, investigators at Dartmouth have observed reactivity of host antibody, in patients entered on their trial, to murine IgM antibodies other than those employed therapeutically (9). Of further interest is the observation that in those reports where the class of host antibody was determined, it appeared to be primarily of the IgG class (Table 3) and that in several clinical investigations, evidence of a host antiglobulin response was detectable within two weeks following initiation of therapy (8,10,13,20).

The rapid kinetics of IgG antiglobulin responses suggests the possibility of a secondary immune response. For this reason, we undertook an in-depth investigation of the host antimouse antiglobulin response in patients receiving monoclonal antibody therapy at the National Cancer Institute (13). Several important observations were made. First, careful analysis with a sensitive solid-phase ELISA assay revealed that small, yet significant, levels of human IgG and IgM reactive with the murine IgG_{2a} antibodies T101 and 9.2.27 could be demonstrated in patients prior to antibody therapy and also in healthy controls (Fig. 1). As depicted in Figure 2, and discussed above, increases in IgG antiglobulin levels could be detected in some patients within two weeks following initiation of treatment. Not surprisingly, patients in the CLL group which demonstrated low levels of antimouse antiglobulin prior to therapy failed to demonstrate elevated levels of antiglobulin following therapy. In examining the specificity of the human antimouse antibody response, we found, as have others, that the specificity of both the preexisting and heightened response was not restricted to the infused antibody. Reactivity was observed with all isotypes of murine IgG, although in our hands little or no reactivity with murine IgM was noted. Only in one case, a melanoma patient treated with the 9.2.27 antibody, did a significant component

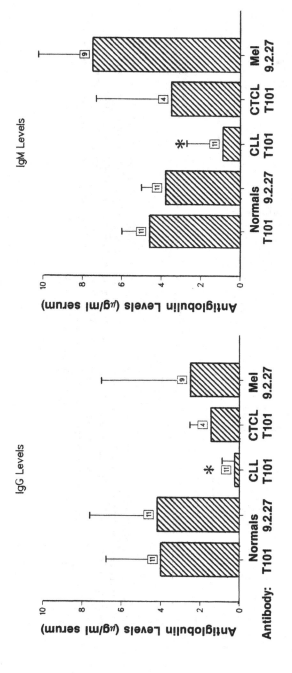

FIGURE 1. Human antimurine IgG reactivity in healthy controls and patients prior to therapy. Serum IgG or IgM antibody levels to both T101 and 9.2.27 antibodies in controls, and the appropriate treatment antibody in patients (T101 for CLL and CTCL patients, 9.2.27 for melanoma patients) are shown. Values represent the mean $\pm$ SD. The number of individuals within each group is indicated over each bar. Levels in patient groups which were significantly lower than those of the appropriate control group ($p < 0.005$ as determined by Student's t-test) are indicated by the * symbol.

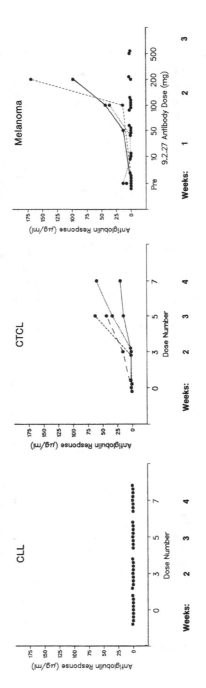

FIGURE 2. Human antimurine IgG levels in 11 CLL, 4 CTCL and 9 melanoma patients. Data points represent determinations on serum specimens obtained either prior to therapy (dose 0) or immediately preceding the indicated dose number or dose level. The number of weeks following initiation of therapy are indicated as a point of reference. Data points connected by lines represent serial specimens from individuals developing an elevated level of human antimurine antibody.

of the antiglobulin response appear to be specific for the infused antibody. In this instance, blocking studies indicated less than 30% inhibition of anti-9.2.27 reactivity when a control murine IgG_{2a} was used as the inhibitor as compared to 90% inhibition when 9.2.27 was used as the inhibitor. Similar studies with sera of other patients indicated 70-90% inhibition of binding to the treatment antibody by any murine immunoglobulin of similar isotype, demonstrating the nonspecific nature of the host antibody. These observations have led us to propose that with the exception of an anti-idiotypic component observed in some patients, the human antimurine immunoglobulin response is largely a secondary immune response. This secondary response is accompanied by elevation of the level of preexisting antiglobulin which is cross-reactive with the mouse antibody administered. Attention must be given, however, to the possibility of a minor anti-idiotypic component in the midst of a greater secondary antiglobulin response.

In addition to the potential for toxicity, of primary importance to the clinical use of monoclonal antibodies is the question of what effect the host antimouse antiglobulin response has upon localization of the monoclonal antibody. In certain instances, antiglobulin responses which have apparently not affected antibody localization have been observed by ourselves (13,21) and others (17). However, the preponderance of evidence indicates that the presence of such antiglobulin in the circulation decreases the ability of the murine antibody to localize on tumor cells, and inhibits further clinical responses in those patients initially responsive (7,8,20). Unique in the literature has been the report by Koprowski and co-workers of patients with gastrointestinal cancer treated with the 17-1A antibody, in which it was hypothesized that human anti-idiotypic antiglobulins elicited by infusion of 17-1A antibody may have been of clinical benefit to the patient (22). In preliminary studies, these investigators have observed a positive correlation between the development of such anti-idiotypic responses and clinical improvements, and they have proposed that the human anti-idiotypic antiglobulin may represent an internal image of the antigen expressed by the tumor cell which is recognized by the infused monoclonal antibody. This internal image may in turn serve as an antigen to induce a host immune response to the antigen expressed by the tumor.

Finally, what steps can be taken to avoid development of a host response to murine immunoglobulin? As described above, studies are underway at the National Cancer Institute to determine whether tolerance can be induced in response to an initially large dose of antibody. Several laboratories have attempted to replace the use of murine monoclonal antibodies with monoclonal antibodies of human origin (23); however, as yet, suitable antibodies have not been developed. Attempts to prevent development of antimouse antiglobulin by drug-induced tolerance with cyclophosphamide have not proven successful (8). The use of plasmapheresis to reduce circulating levels of antibody would not be expected to succeed since attempts to use this technique to reduce plasma antigen levels have not proven successful (19). Even with the limited understanding of how and why human antimouse antiglobulin responses develop, it remains clear that not all individuals develop such a response. It is hoped that investigation will continue into the factors which determine whether an antiglobulin response develops, as well as into identification of procedures capable of identifying those individuals most likely to develop an antiglobulin response.

4. IMMUNE COMPLEX (TYPE III)-MEDIATED REACTIONS TO MONOCLONAL ANTIBODY INFUSION

It is surprising that to date clear evidence for immune complex-mediated clinical reactions in patients treated with monoclonal antibodies has not been seen. Historically, it was immune complex formation that limited the administration of horse antiserum into patients (24). To date, we are aware of only two patients who have had serum sickness-like reactions after monoclonal antibody infusion. Both were patients at the National Cancer Institute who had received escalating intravenous doses of up to 50 or 100 mg of the 9.2.27 monoclonal antibody without complications. Within 10 days after the highest dose, both patients developed skin rashes, headache, low-grade fever, and arthralgia. Renal function was unremarkable in both patients; however, one had minor urinary sediment abnormalities. Both patients immediately responded to corticosteroid adminis- tration and cessation of the 9.2.27 antibody infusion. Other than clinical manifestations, there was no clear evidence for an immune complex-mediated etiology to this syndrome (Fer et al., manuscript in preparation).

In addition, we have observed palpable purpura in one patient 24 hr following T101 monoclonal antibody infusion. It resolved with administration of corticosteroids and cessation of therapy within three days. Palpable purpura is chiefly classified as a leukocytoclastic vasculitis with infiltration of the vessel walls with granulocytes. The exact immune mechanism underlying this phenomenon is not known at this time but is felt to perhaps reflect an immune complex-mediated phenomenon (25).

It is not clear why more immune complex-mediated phenomena have not been observed to date. Perhaps one explanation lies in the nature of the diseases being treated. Although it is clear that some patients with B-cell malignancies treated with anti-idiotype monoclonal antibodies secrete the idiotypic immu- noglobulin into their circulation (19), it would appear that the binding of murine monoclonal antibodies to these circulating antigens does not favor the formation of immune complexes capable of producing clinical disease. This may be because what complexes do form are only transient, or the size of the complexes may not favor the development of the immune complex- mediated tissue injury. Alternatively, murine monoclonal anti- bodies may simply not be capable of activating the human comple- ment cascade. Why circulating immune complexes of the monoclonal antibody and tumor-derived antigens, or the monoclonal antibody and human antiglobulin, do not produce clinically evident immune complex-mediated tissue injury (except in a small number of cases) is not known at this time, but provides another basis for optimism concerning the future clinical uses of murine monoclonal antibodies.

5. CELL-MEDIATED (TYPE IV) IMMUNE REACTIVITY AGAINST MURINE MONOCLONAL ANTIBODIES

As indicated in the introduction, a cell-mediated hypersensitivity reaction is defined as the elicitation of antigen-specific T lymphocytes that migrate to the site of antigenic stimulation, and by direct mechanisms or recruitment of other effector cells, become involved in the elimination of the foreign antigen. Utilizing this narrow definition, it is clear that there is no evidence to date for this type of hypersensitivity reaction in patients receiving monoclonal antibody infusions. The potential reasons for this are probably multifaceted; however, one possible explanation is that murine immunoglobulin belongs to that class of antigens which stimulates humoral immunity more effectively than cell-mediated immunity. Alternatively, it is possible that low levels of antigen-specific T lymphocytes are activated during murine monoclonal antibody therapy, but because of the diffuse systemic distribution of the antibody following infusion, these cells are unable to migrate to one specific area of the body and initiate a focal cell-mediated immune response. While this may be true in the case of leukemias and some types of lymphoma, this is not the case in melanoma. Even though focal sites of tumor exist in these patients, and localization of the administered antibody can be demonstrated, no evidence of a cellular immune response has been demonstrated.

Notable exceptions to this observation are those patients treated with monoclonal antibodies directed against glycolipid melanoma-associated antigens. Antibodies to these antigens are capable of eliciting antibody-dependent cell-mediated cytolysis (ADCC) of target cells in vitro. Cellular influx into tumor sites have been noted in patients treated with these antibodies (26,27). However, these types of responses do not represent classical type IV hypersensitivity responses in that they can be elicited without prior sensitization, and do not appear to involve a memory component since these responses can be observed following the initial course of therapy with a monoclonal antibody.

6. CONCLUSION

We have reviewed our own clinical experiences as well as those of others. It is apparent that several of the reactions which have been observed to monoclonal antibodies do not readily conform to the classical definitions of the four types of hypersensitivity reactions with regard to the hypersensitivity reactions observed in cancer patients receiving murine monoclonal antibodies. However, if these hypersensitivity reactions are examined with regard to their possible pathophysiologic mechanisms, it is clear that the most frequently observed hypersensitivity reaction is the development of anti-murine IgG antibodies (type II immune reactivity). The generation of type II reactivity coupled with circulating foreign antigens can theoretically predispose a patient to the development of immune complex (type III)-mediated hypersensitivity reactions. This may have been the case in the two patients which we observed to develop a serum sickness-like reaction to antimelanoma murine monoclonal antibody therapy, and perhaps explains several of the other forms of toxicity which have been reported thus far. Although the infusion of the T101 monoclonal antibody has been associated with allergic-type clinical symptoms, there has not been any evidence to date that the generation of IgE antibodies is responsible for this phenomenon. Therefore, these hypersensitivity reactions can not be said to be type I (allergic), and may closer resemble type III immune complex-mediated hypersensitivities with tumor and/or normal lymphoid cells forming complexes with the T101 antibody. Finally, there have not been any patients in whom cell-mediated (type IV) hypersensitivity reactions have been observed.

In summary, the types and extent of human immune responses to murine monoclonal antibody infusions have been quite limited. While these few immune responses to the infused antibody have thus far been paralleled by very few clinical responses with the use of murine antibodies alone, the limited host immune responses indicate an excellent potential for murine monoclonal antibodies as targeting agents for drugs, toxins, and radionuclides.

REFERENCES

1. Nadler LM, Stashenko P, Hardy R, et al. 1980. Cancer Res 40:3147.
2. Dillman RO. 1984. CRC Critical Reviews in Oncology/ Hematology 1:357-385.
3. Kashiwagi N, Brantigan C, Buettscheider L, Groth C, Starzly T. 1968. Ann Intern Med 68:275.
4. Royston I, Majda JA, Baird SM, Meserve BL, Griffiths JC. 1980. J Immunol 125:727-731.
5. Foon KA, Schroff RW, Bunn PA, et al. 1984. Blood 64:1085-1093.
6. Foon KA, Schroff RW, Sherwin SA, Oldham RK, Bunn PA, Hsu S-M. 1983. In: Monoclonal Antibodies and Cancer (Eds BD Boss, RE Langman, IS Trowbridge, R Dulbecco), Academic Press, New York, pp 39-52.
7. Dillman RO, Shawler DL, Dillman JB, Royston I. 1984. J Clin Oncol 2:881-890.
8. Miller RA, Oseroff AR, Stratte PT, Levy R. 1983. Blood 62:988-995.
9. Ball ED, Bernier GM, Cornwell GG, McIntyre OR, O'Donnell JF, Fanger MW. 1983. Blood 62:1203-1210.
10. Sears HF, Herlyn D, Steplewski Z, Koprowski H. 1984. J Biol Resp Modif 3:138-150.
11. Sears HF, Mattis J, Herlyn D, et al. 1982. Lancet 1:762-765.
12. Carrasquillo JA, Krohn KA, Beaumier P, et al. Cancer Treat Rep 68:317-328.
13. Schroff RW, Foon KA, Beatty SM, Oldham RK, Morgan AC. 1985. Cancer Res, in press.
14. Foon KA, Schroff RW, Mayer D, et al. 1983. In: Monoclonal Antibodies and Cancer (Eds D Boss, R Langman, I Trowbridge, R Dulbecco), New York, Academic Press, pp 39-52.
15. Ju ST, Cramer DV, Dorf, ME. 1979. J Immunol 123:877-883.
16. Waldmann T, Schroff RW. Unpublished observations.
17. Miller RA, Maloney DG, McKillop J, Levy R. 1981. Blood 58:86-87.
18. Foon KA, Schroff RW, Giardina SL. Unpublished observations.
19. Miller RA, Maloney DG, Warnke R, Levy R. 1982. New Engl J Med 306:517-522.
20. Meeker TC, Lowder J, Maloney DG, et al. 1985. Blood, in press.
21. Oldham RK, Foon KA, Morgan AC, et al. 1984. J Clin Oncol 2:1235-1244.
22. Koprowski H, Herlyn D, Lubeck M, DeFreitas E, Sears HF. 1984. Proc Natl Acad Sci USA 81:216-219.
23. Cote RJ, Morrissey DM, Houghton AN, Beattie EJ, Oettgen HF, Lloyd JO. 1983. Proc Natl Acad Sci USA 80:2026-2030.
24. Steinberg AD, Williams GW. 1976. In: Immunological Diseases (Ed M Sampter), Little, Brown, New York, pp 1530.
25. Sams WM, Claman HN, Kohler PF, McIntosh RM, Small P, Mass, MF. 1975. J Invest Dermatol 64:441.
26. Knuth A, Dippold W, Houghton AN, Meyer zum Buschenfelde KH, Oettgen HF, Old LD. 1984. Proc Am Assoc Cancer Res 25:254.
27. Dippold W, Kunth A, Meyer zum Buschenfelde KH. 1984. Proc Am Assoc Cancer Res 25:247.

7. RADIOLABELED MONOCLONAL ANTIBODIES FOR IMAGING AND THERAPY

JAMES M. WOOLFENDEN and STEVEN M. LARSON

1. INTRODUCTION

The potential of radionuclides for localizing and treating malignant disease has been recognized for decades. A major challenge has been to localize the radionuclides in tumor but not in normal tissue. Although in theory it might be possible to exploit normal physiologic processes to deliver the radionuclides to the tumor, in practice this has been possible in only a few types of cancer. Radioiodine therapy for thyroid carcinoma is the best example of such successful exploitation. Once competing normal thyroid tissue is ablated, differentiated thyroid carcinoma concentrates an administered dose of I-131. The ability of therapeutic doses of I-131 to cure patients with metastatic thyroid carcinoma is well documented (1-3). Other examples of successful therapy with unsealed radionuclides include P-32 for selected cases of polycythemia and thrombocythemia (4) and promising results with I-131-metaiodobenzylguanidine for malignant pheochromocytoma (5).

Lack of a specific delivery system for most tumors has limited the efficacy of radionuclides for tumor localization and has precluded their use for therapy, except in the special cases just noted. Monoclonal antibodies provide the potential for such a specific delivery system. The following review of human studies using radiolabeled monoclonal antibodies for diagnostic imaging and therapy begins with a summary of relevant earlier work using heteroantisera containing antitumor antibodies and concludes with a consideration of problems and prospects for future applications of radiolabeled monoclonal antibodies.

K.A. Foon and A.C. Morgan, Jr. (eds.), *Monoclonal Antibody Therapy of Human Cancer.* Copyright © 1985. Martinus Nijhoff Publishing, Boston. All rights reserved.

2. EARLY ANIMAL STUDIES

The first report of radiolabeled antibody use by Pressman and Keighley in 1948 demonstrated that I-131-labeled anti-rat-kidney globulin localized in rat kidney, but a similarly prepared and labeled anti-albumin did not (6). In a subsequent experiment, rabbit heteroantisera to a murine sarcoma were labeled with I-131 and localized in the mouse tumors, while control rabbit globulin, obtained from the same rabbits before they were immunized, did not (7). Pressman and co-workers later devised an elegant double label technique to follow immune and nonimmune globulin in the same animals simultaneously (8). Purification of tissue-specific antibody was an early problem, but tumor-localizing antibodies could be partially separated from kidney- and liver-localizing antibodies by absorbing the unwanted antibodies with sediments of the tissues to which they bound in vivo (7). Other investigators (9) absorbed kidney-seeking antibody with kidney tissue, eluted the bound antibody, and demonstrated improved kidney uptake of the purified antibody. They also noted that antibody binding to a tissue in vitro did not necessarily predict that the same antibody would do so in vivo.

Many of the problems encountered in the early animal studies remain relevant to contemporary studies using radiolabeled monoclonal antibodies. Animal studies do not always completely predict the biodistribution of antibodies in humans, antibodies may localize in nontumor sites, and adequate control studies are still appropriate to assess whether antibody localization in tumor is actually a tumor-specific process.

3. HUMAN TUMOR LOCALIZATION USING RADIOLABELED HETEROANTISERA

The first human studies of tumor detection and localization using radiolabeled antibodies depended on immunized animals as sources of antibody. Animals such as rabbits, goats, and sheep were immunized with the tumor to be detected. Antibodies were harvested, purified, radiolabeled, and administered to patients. In one of the earliest clinical studies, radiolabeled rabbit antibody to human gliomas appeared promising for tumor localization on rectilinear brain scans (10). Goat antibody to human renal cell carcinoma localized primary tumors in 6 of 7 patients (11) and localized metastases in 6 of 6 patients (12). Antibodies to the animal source of the heteroantisera were encountered in some patients. Two melanoma patients who had previously received either rabbit or goat antimelanoma serum had falsely negative or equivocal scans using radiolabeled heteroantisera from the same source, and they both were found to have circulating anti-rabbit or antigoat antibodies (13).

In 1978 Goldenberg (14) reported very encouraging results using goat antibody to carcinoembryonic antigen (CEA) for radio-immunodetection of a diverse group of human cancers. Eighteen patients were studied; 10 of 11 primary sites were identified, as were 24 of 29 metastatic sites. Imaging involved subtracting the distributions of Tc-99m human serum albumin and Tc-99m pertechnetate from the distribution of I-131 antibody. Circulating CEA levels had no apparent correlation with tumor detection, nor did high levels inhibit tumor detection. Similar studies with sheep anti-CEA using the same subtraction technique identified 4 of 5 primary sites and 8 of 11 metastases (15).

Less encouraging results were reported by Mach (16) using goat anti-CEA and the subtraction method of Goldenberg. He found 11 of 27 colorectal sites to be positive on the unsubtracted images; the subtraction technique made the abnormalities clearer but identified no additional tumor sites. Some labeled antibody activity was present at an additional 8 sites, but the scans would not have been called positive without prior information on tumor location; subtraction did not help at these sites. The final 8 sites were negative on both subtracted and unsubtracted images. Three of the 27 studies were done with labeled F(ab')$_2$ fragments rather than whole antibody; faster tumor localization and less nonspecific liver activity were noted with F(ab')$_2$ as compared to whole immunoglobulin.

Goldenberg and colleagues, using goat antisera and the subtraction techniques noted above, evaluated 25 patients using
I-131 antihuman chorionic gonadotrophin (17). They reported a
sensitivity of 100% (except for one false negative liver metastasis with a true positive primary site) for detecting tropho-
blastic and germinal tumors as well as two cases of lung cancer.
Using I-131 anti-alpha-fetoprotein (AFP), they reported identifying all known tumor sites in 4 patients with hepatocellular
or germ cell tumors; in 8 additional patients with AFP-negative
tumors the labeled anti-AFP showed some uptake in 5 of 19 known
tumor sites, although uptake was less than at AFP-positive
sites (18). Circulating AFP levels up to 15,000 ng/ml did not
appear to interfere with imaging. Other investigators used
sheep anti-AFP in 11 patients and reported similar results
(19).

4. HUMAN STUDIES WITH RADIOLABELED MONOCLONAL ANTIBODIES

Since the early studies of Pressman there had been attempts
to purify antitumor antisera to improve tumor specificity. The
landmark work of Köhler and Milstein (20) in the hybridoma
technology of monoclonal antibodies provided a method for
producing highly purified antibodies.

Diagnostic imaging studies of colorectal cancer were among
the first in vivo clinical applications of radiolabeled monoclonal antibodies. Mach (21) reported some improvement with
monoclonal anti-CEA compared to his earlier work with goat anti-
CEA. In a series of 28 patients, 14 had positive planar images
at 36-48 hours, 6 were equivocal, and 8 were negative. An
additional 14 patients were evaluated using single photon
emission computed tomography (SPECT); primary tumor sites were
correctly identified in 13. However, numerous foci as intense
as the primary tumor sites were noted on the reconstructed SPECT
images and presumably represented reconstruction artifacts.
Another possible cause for false-positive images was the presence
of free iodine, resulting from in vivo deiodination of antibody,
in gastrointestinal tract and bladder, as well as some label in
the reticuloendothelial system. Monoclonal anti-CEA was compared

with nonspecific mouse IgG, and an average ratio of specific to nonspecific tumor uptake of 4.3 was found. In a subsequent multi-institution study using a monoclonal antibody (17-1A) to a cell-bound colorectal carcinoma antigen, sensitivities of 51% with whole antibody and 61% with $F(ab')_2$ fragments in studies of 52 patients with 63 known tumor sites were reported (22). Ratios of tumor activity to adjacent normal tissue ranged from 3.6 to 6.3. Scans using antibody 17-1A and its $F(ab')_2$ fragment were negative in a group of patients with cancers other than colorectal carcinoma.

In another study of monoclonal antibody fragments to colorectal carcinoma antigen, 8 patients with recurrent colon carcinoma involving 32 metastatic sites were studied with $F(ab')_2$ fragments of monoclonal antibody 1083-17-1A (23). Overall lesion detection sensitivity was 69%. Quantitative tumor uptake studies at 48 hours in 3 patients showed from 0.002 to 0.009% of the administered dose per cm^3 of tumor, or from 0.48 to 1.2% of the administered dose in the entire lesion. Tumor to liver ratios rose to an average of 5.6 at 72 hours. They also obtained blood pool images using Tc-99m red blood cells. Blood pool subtraction images were not useful in identifying additional metastatic sites; all lesions could be identified without subtraction. It was concluded that for a site to be called positive, it must be visible on the unsubtracted image, and increased blood pool activity as a possible cause of apparent antibody uptake must be excluded using the blood pool image.

Other investigators (24) used not only antibody 17-1A and its $F(ab')_2$ fragment for detecting colon cancer but also antibody 19.9, which recognizes a tumor-associated sialoganglioside that is shed into the circulation where it can be detected by radioimmunoassay. Antibody 17-1A and its $F(ab')_2$ fragment had a sensitivity of 59% for documented colon cancer sites, and antibody 19.9 and its $F(ab')_2$ fragment had a sensitivity of 66%. When the two antibodies were used together in 12 patients, 10 of 13 tumor sites (77%) were identified.

Malignant melanoma has been an important neoplasm in evaluating radiolabeled monoclonal antibodies for diagnostic imaging and therapy. Melanoma has several well-characterized antigens (25); superficial metastases can be readily evaluated to assess radiolabeled antibody localization for imaging and therapy; and disseminated melanoma cannot be cured with presently available therapy, making an alternative therapy highly desirable. Larson and associates (26,27) evaluated melanoma imaging using I-131-labeled antibodies 96.5 and 8.2 and their Fab fragments; these antibodies are specific for antigen p97, a 97 kilodalton glycoprotein on the melanoma cell surface. In imaging studies of 33 patients using Fab fragments, 20 studies were positive. Ten of the remaining 13 patients had tumors less than 1.5 cm in diameter, 2 had low p97 antigen levels in tumor biopsy specimens, and in 1 patient the Fab iodination was a technical failure. Imaging sensitivity for metastatic sites greater than 1.5 cm diameter was 88%. Twenty patients received simultaneous isotype-matched I-125-Fab not specific for p97; tumor biopsies in 8 of these patients showed specific to nonspecific antibody ratios of approximately 3.5. Antigen concentration was assessed in several of the biopsy specimens using a double determinant radioimmunoassay, and a strong association was noted between p97 concentration and I-131-Fab uptake. An example of antibody imaging is shown in Figure 1. The results of I-131-Fab therapy in these patients will be considered later.

The human imaging studies with radiolabeled monoclonal antibody that have been reviewed thus far all used I-131 as the label. Other similar studies have used I-123 (28). Methods for attaching metals such as indium to proteins using bifunctional chelates have also been described (29,30). Studies using In-111-labeled monoclonal antibodies have been reported in human tumor xenografts in mice (31) and in preliminary human clinical trials (32,33).

PATIENT M.V.
I-131 MoAb (Fab): AP LIVER

p97 SPECIFIC   NON-SPECIFIC   p97 SPECIFIC

 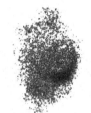 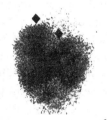

9/30/81 *   11/12/81 *   12/11/81 *

*48 hours post injection

FIGURE 1. Gamma camera images from M.V., a patient with melanoma metastatic to liver. A dose of 4 mCi I-131-(anti-p97)-Fab was injected intravenously on 9/30/81. Uptake in the periphery of a large intrahepatic tumor mass was observed at 48 hours (left panel). The solid diamonds indicate the superior margin of the tumor mass; the hollow diamond indicates the superior margin of normal liver tissue. Control I-131-Fab (from monoclonal antibody 1.4, an IgG$_1$ specific for murine leukemia gp 70) was injected on 11/12/81, and no uptake was observed in tumor at 48 hours (center panel). Repeat I-131-(anti-p97)-Fab injection on 12/11/81 again showed tumor localization (right panel); the tumor had enlarged since the first scan. The solid diamonds again indicate the superior tumor margin. I-131 activity in stomach and intestine presumably represents free iodide. (Reproduced with permission of the American Society for Clinical Investigation from J Clin Invest 72:2107.)

The imaging studies reviewed so far were all obtained after intravenous [in one instance, intraarterial (10)] injection of radiolabeled antibody. Lymphoscintigraphy using radiolabeled particles is widely used (34), but there have been few studies of radiolabeled antitumor antibodies administered subcutaneously and thence into the lymphatics. Order (35) administered I-131 rabbit antiferritin intralymphatically to a patient with Hodgkin's disease and noted uptake and retention of antibody in the involved nodes. DeLand (36) reported promising results using lymphoscintigraphy with goat anti-CEA in patients with breast, gastrointestinal, or genitourinary cancer, although surgical confirmation of presence or absence of disease was limited. Thompson (37) used an anti-breast monoclonal antibody for lymphoscintigraphy. The I-131 antibody showed uptake in all palpable axillary nodes that were confirmed to have metastases, as well as in two nonpalpable nodes that proved to be cancerous. One of the tumor-bearing nodes that was positive on lymphoscintigraphy was negative after intravenous injection of labeled antibody.

5. RADIOIMMUNOTHERAPY USING LABELED ANTITUMOR HETEROSERA

The first treatment of a human cancer with radiolabeled antibodies was initiated at the University of Michigan in 1951 (38). Rabbits were immunized with malignant tissue from a patient with widely metastatic melanoblastoma, and rabbit immune globulin was labeled with I-131 and administered to the patient. Complete tumor regression occurred; the patient was killed in an automobile accident 9 years later, and at autopsy there was no evidence of residual neoplasm. However, similar treatment in 13 subsequent melanoma patients demonstrated no evidence of tumor regression or I-131 tumor localization.

Bale and colleagues noted that anti-fibrin antibodies localized in animal tumors (39), and they proceeded to a clinical trial of rabbit I-131 anti-human-fibrinogen (40). Scans localized tumors in 75% of 172 patients with various neoplasms. Twelve terminal patients who had shown high labeled antibody uptake on scan were given therapeutic trials of 100-160 mCi of

I-131-antibody. The therapy was not effective, possibly due to the irregular antibody distribution that was noted on autoradiographs of tumor sections.

Order and associates (41) used rabbit I-131 antiferritin (3 patients) or anti-CEA (2 patients) as part of a multimodality treatment program. Significant I-131-antibody toxicity was not seen, although it is difficult to separate the therapeutic effects of I-131-antibody from the other modalities. The same group (42) reported decreased tumor size in 4 of 5 hepatoma patients treated with 100-157 mCi I-131 as a single therapy. Radiation dose estimates were 1500-2200 rad to tumor, 400-1000 rad to liver, and 110-220 rad whole body dose (43).

6. RADIOIMMUNOTHERAPY USING LABELED MONOCLONAL ANTIBODIES

Larson (27) and Carrasquillo (44) reported their results in treating a series of patients with metastatic melanoma using I-131-Fab fragments of antibodies 96.5 and 8.2, both directed against p97 antigen, and 48.7, which is directed against the melanoma high molecular weight antigen (250 kilodalton). The melanoma patients received 4 to 10 mg Fab; increasing the amount of Fab was noted to decrease nonspecific localization of I-131-Fab. Individual doses of I-131 ranged from 30 to 342 mCi, with cumulative doses from 132 to 861 mCi in a series of 10 patients. Significant toxicity was not seen below cumulative doses of 500 mCi. Above that level, some patients had a 50% drop in neutrophil and platelet counts, reaching a nadir at 3-4 weeks after I-131-Fab and then improving. One patient who received a cumulative dose of 861 mCi had marked marrow depression after his final dose of 342 mCi, but later showed marrow improvement. One other patient who had had persistent neutropenia after chemotherapy showed a transient 50% drop in platelets and a 32% drop in neutrophils after a single 143 mCi therapy dose.

Radiation dose estimates in the melanoma patients per 100 mCi I-131-Fab were 1040 rad to tumor, 325 rad to liver, and 30 rad to marrow, which was the critical organ. The patients had been selected for treatment based on extensive metastatic disease, presence of high antigen levels in the tumor, and localization

studies using diagnostic doses of I-131-Fab. One important con-
clusion from this study was that I-131-Fab, in properly selected
patients, could be repeatedly localized in tumor. An example
of such localization is shown in Figure 2. Seven of the 10
patients in Carrasquillo's report could not be evaluated for
therapeutic response due to low administered I-131-Fab dose or
advanced disease with short survival. Of the remaining 3
patients, one showed clinical response, with reduction in tumor
mass on computed tomography and palpation; one showed stabili-
zation for 3 months of a previously rapidly growing liver metastasis; and one showed no significant response. All 3 patients
ultimately developed high levels of human antimouse antibody
(HAMA); in the 2 patients who had shown clinical response to
I-131-Fab treatment, HAMA precluded further treatment. The Fab
fragments were less immunogenic than whole antibody; after 4
injections of Fab only 47% of a larger population of melanoma

CC: I-131-(anti-p97)-Fab: 48 hrs.
Anterior Chest

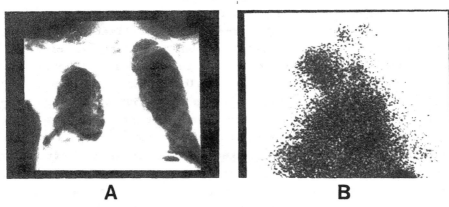

A   B

FIGURE 2. Chest radiograph and anterior chest gamma camera
image from C.C., a patient with melanoma metastatic to lung.
Pulmonary metastases are most prominent radiographically at the
right lung apex and both bases. The gamma camera image was
obtained 48 hours after infusion of 90 mCi I-131-(anti-p97)-Fab
and shows good localization of the therapy dose in tumor,
including prominent mediastinal localization. (Reproduced with
permission from JAMA 249:812.)

patients developed HAMA, compared to 78% after a single whole antibody injection. The main consequence of HAMA was noted to be alteration in antibody biodistribution, with rapid clearance into liver and markedly reduced tumor uptake.

7. PROBLEMS AND PROSPECTS

7.1. Nonspecific labeled antibody distribution

Appropriate control studies are necessary to assess whether tumor uptake of radiolabeled antibodies is actually specific. Tumors typically have expanded extravascular and extracellular space compared to normal tissue; large molecules such as IgG may diffuse in slowly and ultimately reach higher levels than in normal tissues because of this expanded space (45). Bauer (46) noted three decades ago that I-131 albumin localized outside the vascular bed in tumors. The fact that a labeled protein localizes in tumor does not indicate that its uptake is tumor-specific. Pressman (7,8) pioneered the approach of using control globulin to see whether tumor uptake of radiolabeled immune globulin was truly tumor-specific. The same principle should be applied to radiolabeled antitumor monoclonal antibodies, namely comparison with an isotype-matched nonspecific control antibody. Many of the human studies using labeled heteroantisera and some of the studies using labeled monoclonal antibodies lack such controls, and it is difficult to assess their reported results. Moshakis (47) described another method to evaluate specificity of tumor uptake. His "localization index" is the tumor to blood ratio of specific antibody divided by the tumor to blood ratio of nonspecific antibody. Gallagher (48) has discussed these methods and other controls necessary for studies using radiolabeled monoclonal antibodies.

Many workers have used subtraction techniques to attempt to eliminate nonspecific vascular and other background activity. A common method involves subtracting the distributions of Tc-99m pertechnetate and/or Tc-99m albumin or red blood cells from the distribution of labeled antibody. In a statistical evaluation of such methods, Green (49) found that the methods were likely to produce statistical outliers that would be called abnormal,

i.e., false-positive for tumor. A more useful approach to subtraction methods may be that of Moldofsky and associates (23),
who compared labeled antibody images with Tc-99m red blood cell
images to ensure that blood background alone could not account
for apparent antibody uptake. They required that the unsubtracted antibody image show an abnormality, thus preventing
subtraction artifacts from becoming false-positive results.

7.2. Antibody selection and application

Detailed pharmacokinetic comparisons of radiolabeled antitumor whole monoclonal antibody and Fab and F(ab')$_2$ fragments
have not been reported in humans. The fragments are cleared
more rapidly from the blood than whole antibody, and they lack
the nonspecific binding to neutrophils, monocytes, macrophages,
and other cells that is mediated by the Fc portion of the whole
antibody (50). The fragments may be less immunogenic than the
whole antibody (44). Immunogenicity of the fragments is not
trivial, however; I-131-Fab therapy had to be discontinued in 2
patients who had responded due to development of HAMA. Monoclonal
antibodies derived from human-human hybridomas might avoid this
problem (51).

The radiolabeled antibody must be able to find the tumor
antigen. This requires cell surface expression of antigen, as
discussed below. Blood supply to tumor cells is important in
determining whether labeled antibody can find the antigen.
Studies in human tumor xenografts in animals have shown areas
of low antibody uptake caused by decreased blood supply; tissue
sections from such areas, when incubated directly with antibody,
have shown normal antibody uptake, documenting the importance
of tumor blood supply for antibody localization (52).

For certain tumors, administering antibody by routes other
than intravenous may be more effective. Thompson (37) described
monoclonal antibody uptake in a tumor-bearing lymph node with
lymphoscintigraphy but not after intravenous administration of
antibody. We have observed the same phenomenon, and have noted
uptake in nodes outside the expected lymphatic drainage from
the site of injection, perhaps due to trafficking of lymphocytes

labeled in vivo. Intraperitoneal administration of labeled antibody deserves investigation for some abdominal and pelvic tumors.

Carrier antibody may be necessary to saturate circulating antigen or cross-reacting normal tissue antigens. Larson and associates (27) showed that administering unlabeled Fab prior to I-131-Fab greatly diminished nonspecific liver uptake of I-131-Fab, and that liver clearance was saturable in vivo. Dose-response curves evaluating antibody concentration should be obtained for monoclonal antibodies and fragments to determine the optimal antibody dose.

The antibody should have a high affinity for the tumor antigen to help provide good tumor binding. High affinity before labeling does not guarantee high affinity after labeling, since the radiolabeling process may affect antibody immunoreactivity and binding. Ferens (53) found that different antimelanoma Fab fragments had different sensitivity to iodination, as measured by the cell-binding assay. Such postlabeling assays are essential to ensure an immunoreactive product and to determine the best labeling conditions.

7.3. Antigen considerations

True tumor-specific antigens that are constantly expressed on tumor cell surfaces have proved elusive. In one study of breast cancer antigens, Horan Hand (54) found that antigens might be expressed in one area of a tumor but not in another; she also noted a patchwork pattern of alternating antigen-positive and antigen-negative cells. Antigenic expression has been noted to vary in some tumors with cell cycle, reaching a maximum during S-phase (55). This has led to suggestions that synchronizing the cell cycle within a tumor could be useful in radioimmunotherapy (56). Antigenic modulation, the antibody-mediated decrease in expression of target antigen, has been described in several tumor models and has the potential to limit the therapeutic effect of a radiolabeled monoclonal antibody (57). However, antibody-induced modulation of one antigen does not cause modulation of other surface antigens (58). A therapeutic "cocktail" of radiolabeled monoclonal

antibodies directed at more than one antigen might be effica-
cious by decreasing the problem of variable surface antigen
expression and the potential problem of antigenic modulation.
A preliminary study cited earlier noted improved results using
a mixture of two anti-colon-carcinoma antibodies (24).

Lack of antigen specificity has several effects. It contri-
butes to tissue background activity due to nonspecific antibody
binding to nontumor tissue, it may cause false-positive imaging
results, and it may have other clinical consequences. Dillman
(33) noted that 5 of 6 patients who received diagnostic doses
of In-111 monoclonal anti-CEA had marked systemic toxicity and
a 40 to 90% fall in circulating granulocytes, presumably due to
cross-reactivity of the antibody with an antigen on granulocyte
and possibly also erythrocyte cell membranes. He also noted
that the report illustrated one of the limitations of animal
models for assessing monoclonal antibodies, since the effect
had not been observed in an earlier animal study with the same
antibody.

7.4. Radiolabels for imaging

Most of the clinical imaging studies with monoclonal antibodies or fragments have used I-131 as the label. I-131 is
widely available and relatively inexpensive, and iodination
processes have been well described. However, I-131 has several
disadvantages. First, in vivo deiodination occurs and results
in loss of label from the tumor as well as unwanted activity in
thyroid, salivary glands, gastrointestinal tract, and bladder.
Second, the radiation dose associated with beta particle emission, although useful for therapy, limits the administered dose
for diagnostic imaging. Third, the primary gamma emission of
364 KeV is higher than optimal for current nuclear medicine
imaging equipment. A suitable replacement label might have
highly abundant gamma emission(s) in the range of 120-250 keV,
decay by isomeric transition or electron capture, and have a
physical half-life appropriate for the pharmacokinetics of the
antibody being used (perhaps 6 hours to several days).

Indium-111 has been suggested as a promising label, and several early reports of In-111-labeled antibodies have been summarized above. In-111 has a half-life of 2.8 days, decays by electron capture, and has gamma emissions of 171 and 245 keV (88 and 94% abundance, respectively) (59). Tc-99m has excellent physical characteristics (140.5 keV emission of 89% abundance, decay by isomeric transition) although its 6-hour half-life would require rapid blood clearance and tumor uptake for imaging to be practical. I-123 has excellent physical characteristics also (159 keV emission of 83% abundance, decay by electron capture, half-life 13.3 hours), but it has the same problem of _in vivo_ deiodination as I-131. Another possible label might be ruthenium-97 (216 keV, 86%; electron capture; T 1/2 69 hours). The physical properties, advantages, and disadvantages of these radionuclides are summarized in Table 1. Some of the possible labels have been discussed by O'Brien (60). Attaching the labels to monoclonal antibodies or fragments while preserving their immunoreactivity will be a challenge for the radiochemist.

7.5. Radiolabels for therapy

I-131 has been virtually the only radionuclide used for radioimmunotherapy in humans. High level iodination of monoclonal antibodies and fragments has been shown to be feasible (53), and a therapeutic trial using I-131-Fab has already been reviewed. The problem of _in vivo_ deiodination described for imaging applies even more to therapy. An ideal label for therapy should remain on the antibody until it reaches the tumor, remain in tumor tissue through several half-lives, have high linear energy transfer to the target tissue, and lack excessive gamma radiation that poses radiation safety problems for health care personnel. Several alternatives to I-131 have been proposed: other beta particle emitters, Auger electron emitters, and alpha particle emitters.

Copper-67 (Cu-67), a beta emitter, has been evaluated as a candidate label for radioimmunotherapy (61). Cu-67 has a shorter half-life (2.56 vs. 8.04 days) and lower abundance of lower energy gamma emissions than I-131, but the two radionuclides have similar radiation absorbed dose rates per unit activity.

Table 1. Selected radionuclide labels for monoclonal antibody imaging.

Nuclide	Half-life	Decay mode	Gamma energy (abundance)	Advantages	Disadvantages
Iodine-131	8.0 d	B-	364 keV (81%)	Availability Iodine chemistry	Gamma energy In vivo deiodination Radiation dose
Iodine-123	13.3 h	EC	159 keV (83%)	Gamma energy Iodine chemistry	Availability In vivo deiodination
Indium-111	2.8 d	EC	171 keV (88%) 245 keV (94%)	Gamma energy Half-life	
Technetium-99m	6.0 h	IT	141 keV (89%)	Availability Gamma energy	Half-life Chemistry
Ruthenium-97	2.9 d	EC	216 keV (86%)	Gamma energy Half-life	Availability

Physical data are from Lederer (59). Abbreviations: B- = beta emission; EC = electron capture; IT = isomeric transition.

If label is lost from the tumor before several weeks have elapsed, then the shorter half-life of Cu-67 is advantageous for reducing the nontarget radiation dose. The main gamma emission of Cu-67 (185 keV, 47% abundance) is adequate for imaging the distribution of antibody and making radiation dose estimates. Palladium-109 (Pd-109), also a beta emitter, has been chelated using DTPA to a monoclonal antibody to the high molecular weight melanoma antigen and evaluated for therapeutic potential using melanoma xenografts in nude mice (62).

Auger electrons may be useful for radioimmunotherapy. When a radionuclide produces auger electrons (most commonly in association with decay by electron capture or with internal conversion), and when the radionuclide is localized to cells, then the radiation dose to the cells or subcellular components will be considerably greater than predicted by conventional organ or whole body dosimetry (63). This prediction has been confirmed in an animal model comparing radiotoxicity of two radioisotopes of thallium, one decaying by beta particle emission, the other by electron capture; radiotoxicity was greater from the latter due to its associated emission of Auger electrons (64). Intracellular localization of radionuclide may be important for these toxic effects to be observed (65). Jungerman (61) has calculated radiation doses from Auger electron emitters that could be used for radioimmunotherapy. Two examples are mercury-197 (Hg-197) and Pd-100, both of which deposit about 90% of the available energy over a distance of approximately 6 cell diameters; however, Hg-197 has a dose rate that is 3 to 4 times that of Pd-100 and thus would be preferable for therapy.

Several alpha particle emitters have been suggested for therapy or tried in animal models. Astatine-211 (At-211), given intraperitoneally as a radiocolloid, was found to cure experimental malignant ascites in mice, even though P-32 colloid in the same model did not (66). At-211 was noted to have radiations with 1/100th the length but 10 times the linear energy transfer of P-32. Since ionic astatine shares some of the biodistribution characteristics of iodine (67), a stable chemical bond of At-211 to antibody is essential. Bismuth-212 (Bi-212), another alpha emitter, has been suggested as a candidate for therapeutic applications (60). Physical properties of selected radionuclides for radioimmunotherapy are summarized in Table 2. Some of the other possible radionuclides for therapy have been reviewed by O'Brien (60).

8. CONCLUSION

Radiolabeled monoclonal antibodies have been evaluated in humans for localization and treatment of malignant disease. Although the human studies must still be considered preliminary, the results are encouraging. There is still much work to be done. Rigorous studies of labeled antibody pharmacokinetics and application of better labels for imaging and therapy should help to fulfill the promise of these "magic bullets" for cancer diagnosis and treatment.

Table 2. Selected radiolabels for monoclonal antibody radioimmunotherapy.

Nuclide	Half-life	Decay mode	Imaging feasible	Particle maximum energy (abundance)
Iodine-131	8.0 d	Beta	Yes	0.606 MeV (86%)
Copper-67	62.0 h	Beta	Yes	0.577 MeV (20%) 0.484 MeV (35%) 0.395 MeV (45%)
Palladium-109	13.4 h	Beta	No	1.028 MeV (100%)
Yttrium-90	64.1 h	Beta	No	2.288 MeV (100%)
Astatine-211	7.2 h	Alpha	No	5.866 MeV (42%) 7.450 MeV (58%) (from Po-211)
Bismuth-212	60.6 m	Beta 64% Alpha 36%	No	2.251 MeV beta (64%) 1.80 MeV beta complex (36%) (from Tl-208) 6.090 MeV alpha (10%) 6.051 MeV alpha (25%) 8.784 MeV alpha (64%) (from Po-212)
Iodine-125	60.3 d	EC	No	See note
Mercury-197	2.7 d	EC	Marginal	See note
Palladium-100	3.6 d	EC	Marginal	See note
Tin-119	38.0 h	EC	No	See note

Note: Data for Auger and conversion electrons are contained in the report of Jungerman et al. (61). Other physical data are from Lederer (59). EC = electron capture.

157

158

REFERENCES

1. Benua RS, Cicale NR, Sonenberg M, Rawson RW. 1962. Am J Roentgenol 87:171-182.
2. Mazzaferri EL, Young RL. 1981. Am J Med 70:511-518.
3. Beierwaltes WH. 1978. Semin Nucl Med 8:79-94.
4. Chaudhuri TK. 1978. In: Therapy in Nuclear Medicine (Ed RP Spencer), Grune & Stratton, New York, pp 223-235.
5. Sisson JC, Shapiro B, Beierwaltes WH, et al. 1984. J Nucl Med 24:197-206.
6. Pressman D, Keighley G. 1948. J Immunol 59:141-146.
7. Pressman D, Korngold L. 1953. Cancer 6:619-623.
8. Pressman D, Day ED, Blau M. 1957. Cancer Res 17:845-850.
9. Bale WF, Spar IL. 1957. Adv Biol Med Phys 5:285-356.
10. Day ED, Lassiter S, Woodhall B, Mahaley JL, Mahaley MS Jr. 1965. Cancer Res 25:773-778.
11. Belitsky P, Ghose T, Aquino J, Norvell ST, Blair AH. 1978. J Nucl Med 19:427-430.
12. Belitsky P, Ghose T, Aquino J, Tai J, MacDonald AS. 1978. Radiology 126:515-517.
13. Ghose T, Guclu A, Tai J, MacDonald AS, Norvell ST, Aquino J. 1975. Cancer 36:1646-1657.
14. Goldenberg DM, DeLand FH, Kim E, et al. 1978. New Engl J Med 298:1384-1388.
15. Dykes PW, Hine KR, Bradwell AR, et al. 1980. Br Med J 280: 220-222.
16. Mach J-P, Carrel S, Forni M, Ritschard J, Donath A, Alberto P. 1980. New Engl J Med 303:5-10.
17. Goldenberg DM, Kim EE, DeLand FH. 1981. Proc Natl Acad Sci USA 78:7754-7758.
18. Goldenberg DM, Kim EE, DeLand FH, et al. 1980. Cancer 45: 2500-2505.
19. Halsall AK, Fairweather DS, Bradwell AR, et al. 1981. Br Med J 283:942-944.
20. Köhler G, Milstein C. 1975. Nature 256:495-497.
21. Mach J-P, Buchegger F, Forni M, et al. 1981. Immunol Today 2:239-249.
22. Mach J-P, Chatal J-F, Lumbroso J-D, et al. 1983. Cancer Res 43:5593-5600.
23. Moldofsky PJ, Powe J, Mulhern CB Jr, et al. 1983. Radiology 149:549-555.
24. Chatal J-F, Saccavini J-C, Fumoleau P, et al. 1984. J Nucl Med 25:307-314.
25. Hellström KE, Hellström I, Brown, JP. 1984. In: Monoclonal Antibodies and Cancer (Ed GL Wright, Jr), Dekker, New York, pp 31-47.
26. Larson SM, Brown JP, Wright PW, Carrasquillo JA, Hellström I, Hellström KE. 1983. J Nucl Med 24:123-129.
27. Larson SM, Carrasquillo JA, Krohn KA, et al. 1983. J Clin Invest 72:2101-2114.
28. Epenetos AA, Mather S, Granowska M, et al. 1982. Lancet 2:999-1004.
29. Sundberg MW, Sherman DG, Meares CF, Goodwin DA. 1974. J Med Chem 17:1304-1307.

30. Meares CF, Goodwin DA, Leung CSH, et al. 1976. Proc Natl Acad Sci USA 73:3803-3806.
31. Scheinberg DA, Strand M, Gansow OA. 1982. Science 215:1511-1513.
32. Rainsbury RM, Westwood JH, Coombes RC, et al. 1983. Lancet 2:934-938.
33. Dillman RO, Beauregard JC, Sobol RE, et al. 1984. Cancer Res 44:2213-2218.
34. Ege GN. 1983. Semin Nucl Med 13:26-34.
35. Order SE, Bloomer WD, Jones AG, et al. 1975. Cancer 35:1487-1492.
36. DeLand FH, Kim EE, Corgan RL, et al. 1979. J Nucl Med 20:1243-1250.
37. Thompson CH, Lichtenstein M, Stacker SA, et al. 1984. Lancet 2:1245-1247.
38. Beierwaltes WH, Khazaeli MB. 1983. In: Radioimmunoimaging and Radioimmunotherapy (Eds SW Burchiel, BA Rhodes), Elsevier, New York, pp 419-435.
39. Bale WF, Spar IL, Goodland RL. 1960. Cancer Res 20:1488-1494.
40. Spar IL, Bale WF, Marrack D, Dewey WC, McCardle RJ, Harper PV. 1967. Cancer 20:865-870.
41. Order SE, Klein JL, Ettinger D, Alderson P, Siegelman S, Leichner P. 1980. Int J Radiat Oncol Biol Phys 6:703-710.
42. Order SE, Klein JL, Leichner PK. 1981. Oncology 38:154-160.
43. Leichner PK, Klein JL, Garrison JB, et al. 1981. Int J Radiat Oncol Biol Phys 7:323-333.
44. Carrasquillo JA, Krohn KA, Beaumier P, et al. 1984. Cancer Treat Rep 68:317-328.
45. Bale WF, Contreras MA, Grady ED. 1980. Cancer Res 40:2965-2972.
46. Bauer FK, Tubis M, Thomas HB. 1955. Proc Soc Exp Biol Med 90:140-142.
47. Moshakis V, McIlhinney RAJ, Raghavan D, Neville AM. 1981. J Clin Pathol 34:314-319.
48. Gallagher BM. 1983. In: Animal Models in Radiotracer Design (Eds RM Lambrecht, WC Eckelman), Springer-Verlag, New York, pp 61-105.
49. Green AJ, Begent RJH, Keep PA, Bagshawe KD. 1984. J Nucl Med 25:96-100.
50. Dorrington KJ, Painter RH. 1977. In: Progress in Immunology III (Ed TE Mandel), North Holland, New York, pp 298-305.
51. Kaplan HS, Olsson L. 1982. In: Hybridomas in Cancer Diagnosis and Treatment (Eds MS Mitchell, HF Oettgen), Raven Press, New York, pp 113-132.
52. Moshakis V, McIlhinney RAJ, Neville AM. 1981. Br J Cancer 44:663-669.
53. Ferens JM, Krohn KA, Beaumier PL, et al. 1984. J Nucl Med 25:367-370.
54. Horan Hand P, Nuti M, Colcher D, Schlom J. 1983. Cancer Res 43:728-735.
55. Kufe DW, Nadler L, Sargent L, et al. 1983. Cancer Res 43:851-857.

56. Burchiel SW. 1983. In: Radioimmunoimaging and Radioimmuno-
    therapy (Eds SW Burchiel, BA Rhodes), Elsevier, New York,
    pp. 14-23.
57. Shawler DL, Miceli MC, Wormsley SB, Royston I, Dillman RO.
    1984. Cancer Res 44:5921-5927.
58. Ritz J, Pesando JM, Notis-McConarty J, Schlossman SF. 1980.
    J Immunol 125:1506-1514.
59. Lederer CM, Shirley VS, eds. 1978. Table of Isotopes, 7th
    ed, Wiley, New York.
60. O'Brien HA Jr. 1983. In: Radioimmunoimaging and Radioimmuno-
    therapy (Eds SW Burchiel, BA Rhodes), Elsevier, New York,
    pp 161-169.
61. Jungerman JA, Yu K-HP, Zanelli CI. 1984. Int J Appl Radiat
    Isot 35:883-888.
62. Fawwaz RA, Wang TST, Srivastava SC, et al. 1984. J Nucl Med
    25:796-799.
63. Wrenn ME, Howells GP, Hairr LM, Paschoa AS. 1973. Health
    Phys 24:645-653.
64. Rao DV, Govelitz GF, Sastry KSR. 1983. J Nucl Med 24:145-
    153.
65. Kassis AI, Adelstein SJ, Haydock C, Sastry KSR. 1983.
    J Nucl Med 24:1164-1175.
66. Bloomer WD, McLaughlin WH, Neirinckx RD, et al. 1981.
    Science 212:340-341.
67. Brown I, Carpenter RN, Mitchell JS. 1984. Int J Appl Radiat
    Isot 35:843-847.